Dr Russ Harris is a world expert on ACT, a new mindfulness-based approach to psychological change that is rapidly sweeping this country. In the last four years, Russ has trained over 8,000 coaches, counsellors and psychologists in this model, which enables people to reduce stress, overcome fear and find fulfilment. He has written four books, including the hugely successful self-help title *The Happiness Trap* (2007), now published in twenty countries and fifteen languages. A popular speaker, Russ runs ACT training all over Australia and internationally, and from July 2011 he will be running ACT workshops for the general public.

THE CONFIDENCE GAP

Dr Russ Harris

ROBINSON

ROBINSON

First published by 2010 by Penguin Group (Australia)

First published in Great Britain in 2011 by Robinson
Reprinted in 2019 by Robinson

1 3 5 7 9 10 8 6 4 2

A CIP catalogue record for this book
is available from the British Library.

ISBN 978-1-4721-4447-8

Printed and bound in Great Britain by Clays Ltd, Elcograf S.p.A.

Papers used by Robinson are from well-managed forests
and other responsible sources

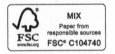

Robinson
An imprint of
Little, Brown Book Group
Carmelite House
50 Victoria Embankment
London EC4Y 0DZ

An Hachette UK Company
www.hachette.co.uk

www.littlebrown.co.uk

To Yulanie and Bruce

Thank you both so much for all your love, support and
encouragement; for gently showing me the way when
I wandered off; for being there when I needed
you; and for bringing so much warmth
and light into my life.

contents

how lucky is that?

foreword by Steven Hayes

It is hard to be a human being. We are perhaps more challenged than any other creature on the planet.

'That's ridiculous,' comes the retort. 'Look around you. In the developed world, at least, we have everything we need: food, water, safety, warmth, shelter, social stimulation.' That is true, but it only makes the human condition all the more poignant. How can it be that the same creatures who have everything, relatively speaking, also worry about the future, ruminate over past failures, or feel crushed by their fears and self-doubts?

The answer is rather surprising. The exact same abilities that lead to our successes lead to our struggles.

The human mind is a problem-solving organ. It detects dangers, analyses situations, predicts outcomes and suggests actions. In the world outside our skins, that works wonderfully well. But when those same logical abilities are turned within, a human life becomes a problem to be solved rather than a process to be experienced. A trap opens up. Life gets put on hold while we fight a war within.

There is a simple reason for this. The world within is not logical, it's psychological.

The rules of human growth and experience are almost the exact opposite of those in the external world. When there is a smelly piece of food lying on the floor, throwing it out into the dustbin works perfectly well. That exact same action is horribly ineffective when applied to our deepest fears.

If you at this moment are caught in an intense struggle with self-confidence you are profoundly lucky. Profoundly. Life has dealt you a winning hand. Let me explain.

Most people dealing with confidence issues are living life like a person with their foot caught in a heavy animal trap. Most will think the problem is with them, not the trap they happened to step into. They will hobble down the street in pain, slowed down by the trap.

Maybe that is rather like where you are right now. So why are you lucky? Well, for one thing, you know your foot is ensnared. Many who are caught in this trap do not. They just slog on, trying to ignore the pain.

You are also lucky because you have in your hands a scientifically proven method of springing the trap. Many others will desperately try out the usual hokum that modern science now knows will almost certainly not set them free.

And you are lucky because if you learn how to deal with confidence problems, you will be far, far better prepared to cope with other problems that work the same way if (or more realistically, when!) they grab you. Your suffering was the price of admission, but it has already been paid. Enough is enough. Now it is time for the challenging fun of learning and transformation.

It is going to be a heck of a lot more joyful to move ahead in life without dragging those heavy, hurtful traps around with you wherever you go.

Fortunately, the book you are holding is going to help you see precisely where the gap lies between a lack of self-confidence and doing things that will work. And if you give this book a chance you are likely to find a psychologically workable way forward.

That last statement is not a guarantee – it is a prediction. Russ does not talk very much about the science underlying this work, but it is voluminous and growing. The basic science of mind you see in these pages covers at least 150 studies, and is indirectly supported by hundreds more. They all show that most people who read these books improve significantly, provided that they read them carefully and practise their methods.

In this brilliant book, he shows us exactly how the gap forms and teaches us the rules for human growth and transformation. Russ is perhaps the clearest writer in the Acceptance and Commitment Training (ACT) universe, and one of the most gifted clinicians and talented trainers. He has an amazing ability to make the complex seem simple. And he has done it yet again in this volume. I've been working on ACT for thirty years and I'm sitting here and I'm feeling deeply moved, energized and schooled. Russ has opened my eyes. *Again*.

If you could be released from your struggle with self-confidence, wouldn't you consider yourself lucky? If you could learn something profound that would be of use to you in the rest of your life wouldn't you thank the fates that gave you the keys to that more liberated path?

On the other side of your struggle, you may come to see the words I began this with differently: It is hard to be a human being. It is not hard because we have few resources, or because horrific things happen to us, even though sadly that occurs. It is hard for us all because it is tricky to have our logical minds – the source of our greatest strength and achievement – so seductively invite us into a trap.

You are about to learn how to respectfully decline that invitation.

How lucky is that?

Peace, love and life,

Steven C. Hayes

Professor of Psychology, University of Nevada

Author of *Get Out of Your Mind and Into Your Life*

30,000 feet over the Midwestern skies

5 June 2010

introduction

a daring adventure, or nothing

If only you had more confidence, how would your life be different?

Whether you call it 'lack of confidence', 'fear of failure', 'performance anxiety' or 'self-doubt', the chances are it's cost you dearly in your life. Take a moment to consider: what have you given up? What have you missed out on? What opportunities have you lost because of it?

Over the years, I've worked with literally thousands of people who have put their hopes, dreams and ambitions on hold because they 'don't have enough confidence'. And the sad thing is, this lack of confidence is not due to any fault of their own. It is certainly not because of stupidity, or laziness, or negative thinking, or a deprived childhood, or a chemical imbalance in the brain. It is simply because they do not know the rules of the confidence game.

THE CONFIDENCE GAME

Yes, confidence is a game – a skilful psychological game. And unfortunately, our society gives us the wrong rules to play it. Over the years you may have read articles, bought self-help books, watched TV shows and listened to well-meaning advice from friends, family and health professionals on how to overcome fear of failure, eliminate self-doubt or boost self-confidence. And I'd guess that some of those ideas worked quite well – at least, for a little while. But I'd also be willing to bet that they didn't ultimately give you what you wanted. So, are you open to something new? Something challenging? Are you willing to try playing with a radically different set of rules?

I'm not going to churn out the same old stuff you've heard a million times before: vizualisation, self-hypnosis, positive affirmations, challenging negative thoughts, relaxation techniques, self-esteem boosting, 'fake it till you make it' strategies and so on. Nor will I deny reality and claim that you can have anything you want simply through asking the universe and believing it will provide. (Of course, I'd sell a lot more books that way – nothing sells as well as promising you can have whatever you want for virtually no effort!)

Instead, I'll show you why it's not your fault that what you've been trying isn't working. Until now, you may have thought that you weren't trying hard enough, or you weren't 'doing it properly': that you weren't thinking positively enough, or challenging your negative thoughts effectively enough, or practising your relaxation techniques/self-hypnosis/visualization intensively enough, etc. But you'll soon realise that while these popular strategies can often give us relief from fear, anxiety and self-doubt in the short term, they rarely give us genuine confidence in the long term. Why not? Because they are based on the wrong rules for the confidence game. And there's no way to win the game if you don't know the rules!

Now just for a moment, stop reading and notice what thoughts you are having. Throughout this book, I'll be asking you to do this repeatedly: to increase your awareness of what your mind is doing; to notice how it's reacting and what it's telling you. The ability to notice your own thought processes is an important psychological skill. And the more often you do this, the more you will learn about how your mind works – which will come in very handy later. So please, just for a few seconds, put the book down and simply notice what your mind is telling you.

***

Are you noticing thoughts such as: 'How did this happen? Where did I go wrong? How did I come to learn the "wrong rules"'? The truth is, it's almost impossible that you could have grown up in our modern society without learning these rules. You've been learning them since you were a tiny kid. They are deeply entrenched and widely promoted through popular myths, Hollywood movies, glossy magazines, pop psychologists, self-help gurus, hypnotherapists, motivational speakers and the 'common sense' advice that we so frequently receive from professionals, friends and relatives.

It's clinging to these rules tightly that keeps many people firmly stuck in the 'confidence trap'. They keep trying to overcome fear and boost self-confidence using tools and strategies that are only effective for a short time, and keep them constantly striving for 'more confidence'.

So what are all these 'wrong rules'? And more importantly, what are the 'right rules' to help us win the confidence game? As you read through this book, you'll progressively find out. I don't want to lay it all out for you right now, before we've even reached the first chapter. Rather, I invite you to treat this book as an adventure; a voyage of discovery. I encourage you to savour the process of exploration, and to enjoy each new encounter along the way. On your journey, you'll discover a revolutionary new approach to maximizing human potential: a model of change which is firmly based on cutting-edge research in human psychology. And you'll learn to develop a mindset known as psychological flexibility – a powerful mental state that enables you to respond effectively to fear, anxiety and self-doubt. You'll also learn to develop genuine, lasting self-confidence. And you'll learn to enhance your performance in any area of life – from sports, business and creative arts to socialising, parenting and sex!

TOO GOOD TO BE TRUE?

If at this point you're feeling doubtful or cynical, I think that's good – and I'd encourage you to maintain your scepticism. Please, do *not* believe anything just because I say it's so. After all, if 'believing what others tell you' were the best way to resolve your problems, you'd have sorted them out long ago. So rather than automatically believing what I say, please always check your own experience and see if it is true for you.

Can I absolutely guarantee that the methods in this book will work for you? Well, if you ever encounter anyone who makes you a foolproof guarantee of success, then please – do not buy anything they are offering. A guarantee of this nature is a sure sign of insincerity (or self-delusion). Even a top surgeon would never guarantee that an operation would be a total success. He would tell you his best estimate of the odds of success, and then he'd get you to sign a consent form acknowledging the small but possible risks of all the things that might go wrong.

So what are your odds of success if you use the methods in this book? Very, very high. Why do I say that? Because this book is based upon a new model for changing human behaviour that is shaking the very foundations of Western psychology. In the worlds of sport and business, this model has various names, including the Mindfulness-Acceptance-Commitment Approach, Mindfulness-based Emotional Intelligence Training, or Psychological Flexibility Training. Most commonly it is known as Acceptance and Commitment Training, or ACT (which is said as the word 'act', not as the initials A-C-T).

US psychologist Professor Steven Hayes developed ACT in the early 1980s, originally to treat depression. (In the world of counselling and psychotherapy, it is known as Acceptance and Commitment *Therapy*.) Unfortunately, back then ACT was such a revolutionary concept, it took more than twenty-five years before the wider world of psychology was able to embrace its insights. Now, as ever more evidence accumulates to prove its effectiveness, ACT is rapidly spreading around the globe, having a powerful impact on many difficult areas of people's lives. And one key factor in its success is its innovative approach to developing mindfulness.

WHAT IS MINDFULNESS?

Mindfulness is a mental state of awareness, openness and focus. When we are mindful, we are able to engage fully in what we are doing, let go of unhelpful thoughts, and act effectively without being pushed around by our emotions. Mindfulness has been known about in Eastern philosophy for thousands of years, but until recently we in the West could only learn about it through following ancient doctrines from the East such as yoga, meditation, tai chi, martial arts or Zen. ACT allows us to develop mindfulness skills in a short space of time, even if we don't follow these ancient traditions.

There are three key mindfulness skills that will play a major role in your journey to genuine confidence. These are known as defusion, expansion and engagement.

Defusion
Defusion is the ability to separate from your thoughts and to let them come and go, instead of getting caught up in them, or allowing them to dictate what you do. Defusion provides a powerful way to deal effectively with painful, unhelpful or self-defeating thoughts and beliefs.

Expansion
Expansion is the ability to open up and make room for emotions, sensations and feelings, and to let them come and go without letting them drag you down, push you around or hold you back. Expansion provides a powerful way to handle difficult emotions such as fear, anger and anxiety.

Engagement
Engagement is the ability to be 'psychologically present'; to live fully 'in the moment'; to be fully aware of what is happening right here, right now, instead of being caught up in your thoughts; to be open to, curious about and actively involved in your here-and-now experience. Engagement is an essential ability if you wish to perform well, or find satisfaction and fulfilment in whatever you are doing.

BUT THERE'S MORE
There's more to ACT than developing mindfulness skills; it also involves clarifying your core values – your heart's deepest desires for how you want to behave as a human being – and using those values to motivate, inspire and guide your ongoing action. When

mindfulness, values and committed action come together, they give rise to 'psychological flexibility': the ability to take effective action, guided by values, with awareness, openness and focus.

The ACT model is remarkable in its adaptability. The same tools that have helped tens of thousands of people worldwide to reclaim, rebuild and enrich their lives after many years of struggling with drug addiction, alcoholism, depression, panic disorder and schizophrenia are now being used to help professional athletes and businesspeople enhance their performance, to enable organizations to run more effectively, and to help all sorts of workers – from police officers and bankers to receptionists and dentists – to reduce stress and increase satisfaction in their work. In this book you will discover how to use those tools to develop genuine confidence, pursue your dreams and be the person you really want to be. But first let me tell you a little bit about myself.

MY STORY

Confidence is a topic that's very close to my heart, because for many, many years I didn't have it! As a teenager and in my twenties, I was incredibly anxious in social situations, full of self-doubt and terrified of coming across as dull, stupid or unlikeable. Long before I reached the legal drinking age, I started relying on alcohol to help me cope, and by the end of my first year at medical school, I was drinking heavily on a daily basis. This got progressively worse, and on one occasion, in my third year at medical school, I was admitted to hospital, via ambulance, with alcohol poisoning. (My embarrassment was intense, but not as bad as the hangover.)

My low self-confidence also played out in intimate relation-ships. I was so afraid of rejection, I never asked girls to go out with me unless I was drunk – and they usually only said 'yes' if they were drunk too! On those rare occasions when I did actually have a girlfriend, I would usually end the relationship after two weeks.

I figured if I ended it quickly, she wouldn't get a chance to realize how 'inadequate' I was; in other words, I got to reject her before she could reject me.

I had similar problems with studying. At medical school, I was convinced that I was more stupid than everyone else in my year, and whenever I tried to plough my way through all those thick, complex textbooks of anatomy, physiology and biochemistry, all my self-doubt came gushing to the surface. So what did I do? Well, I didn't like those feelings of anxiety, or those thoughts about being stupid, so to avoid them, I avoided studying! And the consequence? For my first two years at medical school, I failed every single exam, and had to resit them all. (Of course, the heavy drinking didn't help.)

I was very lucky I didn't get thrown out of medical school; at the time, I set a new record for failing exams. I always managed to do just enough work to pass them on the resits. Eventually, I learned my lesson. In my fourth year at medical school, I started to study sensibly, and two years later, I qualified as a doctor. Which gave me a huge sense of achievement. But did that boost my low self-confidence?

Far from it!

Once I had graduated, my self-doubt went through the roof. Working as a junior hospital doctor, I was constantly in a state of high anxiety. I was terrified of making the wrong decision, or giving the wrong drug, or missing the correct diagnosis. My hands always get sweaty when I'm nervous – but at this point in my life, they weren't so much sweating as dripping. I would wipe them dry on the sides of my white coat, but within moments they would be hot and clammy again. And if I had to wear rubber gloves for medical procedures, the gloves would literally fill up with sweat. After a few weeks of this relentless sweating, I developed a nasty case of dermatitis: my fingers erupted into a mass of red blisters and required treatment with steroids to settle down.

So I know what it's like to lack self-confidence. I've given up on many things that were important to me. I've missed out on important areas of life. I've held myself back through self-doubt and fear of failure. And the good news is, I've been able to learn and change. These days I socialize with confidence – but hardly drink at all. I study with confidence – and then go on to write books about what I learn. I work with confidence – which includes speaking to audiences all over the world. So I trust the principles in this book not only because they are solidly backed by science, not only because I have witnessed them helping hundreds of my clients, but because they have worked so well for me in *my* life.

THERE'S NO SUCH THING AS A FREE LUNCH

If you're open to new ideas and willing to learn some new skills, then the odds are overwhelming that you'll be successful in developing genuine confidence. However, not surprisingly, like everything that improves your life, this will take time and effort. You'll need to invest time and effort not only to read this book, but also to practise these new skills and apply them in the relevant areas of your life. Take a moment to think about whether you're prepared to invest that time and energy.

We wouldn't expect to become a good skier or painter or dancer simply by reading books about it. Reading books about these subjects can give us plenty of valuable information, but in order to ski well, paint well, dance well, we actually need to practise the relevant skills. And the same holds true for developing genuine confidence. This book will give you both the tools you need and the instructions for using them – but you'll need to do some practice to reap the benefits. (And if you're feeling a sense of reluctance or hesitation – if your mind's saying something like 'But I don't have the discipline/motivation/willpower' – not to worry; those are all issues we'll cover in this book.)

SO WHERE TO FROM HERE?

This book is structured in five parts. Part 1 is called 'Warming Up'. Here, I'll be challenging some popular myths around confidence, and you'll discover how we all learned to play by the wrong rules. In part 2, 'The Double-Edged Sword' you'll learn how to effectively handle those negative thoughts that all of us have (without disputing them or trying to replace them with positive affirmations, and so on). In part 3, 'What Gets You Going', you'll discover the fundamentals of self-motivation and how to overcome psychological barriers. In part 4, 'Taming Your Fear', you'll learn, step by step, how to fundamentally transform your relationship with fear and anxiety. And in part 5, 'Playing the Game', you'll discover how to bring all your new skills together for genuine confidence, ongoing success and peak performance in your chosen field of endeavour.

At school, you probably learned about Helen Keller. Born in 1880, Helen was nineteen months old when she was struck by meningitis, which left her permanently deaf and blind. Against all the odds, she learned to read and write, and went on to become a great author, a powerful advocate for progressive social change, and ultimately a Nobel prize-winner. She is widely quoted in countless books, and probably her most famous saying is this: 'Life is a daring adventure, or nothing.'

Given these two options for your life – a daring adventure, or nothing – which do you choose? If you want your life to be a daring adventure; if you want to grow, explore and develop your full potential; if you're ready now to set out in a brave new direction, curious about what you will discover, and willing to make room for the discomfort that may arise . . . then what are you waiting for?

part one

warming up

chapter 1

why bother?

So what's in this book for you?

On one level, the answer is obvious: you want more confidence. But I want you to dig a bit deeper, because confidence is not the end of the journey, is it? Presumably you want that confidence in order to achieve something: to make changes that will improve your life.

Imagine that you magically have all the confidence you ever could have hoped for – but nothing in your life changes. You feel supremely confident, but you continue to act in exactly the same way as before, in every aspect of your life. There are no changes in your relationships, your work, your health, your social life or your recreational activities. You continue to go through the same old daily routine, doing the same old things. You walk and talk exactly as before. You don't start any new projects. You don't pursue any new goals. Your performance doesn't alter in any way. Your character doesn't change. You don't treat yourself or others any differently. You behave in exactly the same way as you did before.

13

The only thing different is that you now feel confident. Would you be satisfied with that outcome?

I've asked hundreds of people that question, and no one has ever answered 'yes'. This is hardly surprising. We don't want confidence just for the sake of it; we want it for a purpose. We want it to help us achieve our goals, follow our dreams or perform better in some domain of life, such as sport, business, music, the arts, public speaking, parenting or socializing. That's why I ask my clients, 'If you had all the confidence in the world, how would you behave differently? What sort of person would you be and what sort of things would you do?'

The answers I get to this question vary enormously. Below, I'll give you just a small sample.

- Dave, a fifty-year-old physiotherapist, would be more creative, and start writing that novel he's been dreaming about for over a decade.
- Claire, a somewhat shy thirty-three-year-old receptionist who hasn't been out on a date in more than four years, would join an online dating agency and start meeting some new people. She would also become more outgoing, open and talkative both at the office and amongst her friends.
- Ethan, a senior manager in a large corporation, would be more effective at making decisions under pressure and better at giving performance appraisals to his staff.
- Raj, the owner of a very successful restaurant, would take out a loan and open the second restaurant he's been dreaming about for over two years.
- Koula, an insurance-claims processor, would leave her empty, joyless marriage and start a new relationship.
- Rob, a forty-two-year-old real estate agent looking for

a change in career, would enrol part-time at university and start studying for his MBA.

- Sarah, an unemployed dancer, would attend far more auditions and dance much better in front of the judges.
- Phil, a semi-professional tennis player, would play better under pressure – and hopefully win more games as a result.
- Cleo, a shy twenty-eight-year-old scientist, would make more friends, spend more time socializing, and behave in a more genuine, warm and engaging way in social situations.
- Seb, a forty-four-year-old taxi driver, would start making love to his wife again. For the past three years, he has avoided all sexual activity for 'fear of failure'.
- Dana, a junior manager in a large manufacturing company, would contribute more in meetings, including sharing her genuine opinions and giving suggestions.
- Alexis, a twenty-eight-year-old mother of two young boys, would be more assertive with her domineering, hypercritical mother-in-law.

Now you've had a glimpse of other people's desires, it's time to connect with your own. Please take as long as you need to read through and carefully consider the important questions that follow.

In a world where you had unlimited confidence:

- How would you behave differently?
- How would you walk and talk differently?
- How would you play, work and perform differently?
- How would you treat others differently: your friends, relatives, partner, parents, children and work colleagues?
- How would you treat yourself differently?
- How would you treat your body?

- How would you talk to yourself?
- How would your character change?
- What sort of things would you start doing?
- What would you *stop* doing?
- What goals would you set and work towards?
- What difference would your new-found confidence make in your closest relationships, and how would you behave differently around those people?
- What difference would your new-found confidence help you to make in the world?

***

Please take some time to reflect on these questions before reading on. Get clear about the purpose underlying your quest for more confidence. Your answers to these questions are vitally important; they will provide the values and goals for your ongoing journey. And because so many people are unclear about the difference between values and goals, let's take a few moments to quickly explore it.

VALUES AND GOALS

Values are 'desired qualities of ongoing action'. In other words, your values describe how you want to behave as a human being: how you want to act on an ongoing basis; what you want to stand for in life; the principles you want to live by; the personal qualities and character strengths you want to cultivate. For example, common values in intimate relationships include trust, honesty, openness, integrity, equality, respect, and being loving, caring, supportive and assertive. These are all qualities of action, ways of behaving throughout your life. Values can never be completed or ticked off the list as 'done'; they are ongoing. If you value being

16

loving in your relationship, there never comes a time when being loving is completed.

Goals are 'desired outcomes'. In other words, goals are what you want to get, complete, possess or achieve. Goals are *not* ongoing. The moment you achieve a goal, you can tick it off the list; it is over, completed, 'done'.

So suppose you want to have a great job: that's a goal. The moment you get that job, goal achieved. But suppose you want to be effective, efficient and productive; to engage fully in your work and pay careful attention to what you are doing; to be open, friendly and caring towards others in the workplace. Those are values, not goals; they are how you want to behave throughout your life.

And notice you can live by these values even if you *never* get that great job. If these values are truly important to you, you can choose to live by them in any job you do, from waiting on tables to running a multinational company. (You can also live by them in unpaid jobs, such as rearing your kids.)

You can think of values as a compass: you use them to set a direction, and help you stay on track during the journey. But looking at a compass won't give you a journey. The journey only starts when you take action.

Acting on your values is like travelling west. No matter how far west you travel, there's always further to go; you never reach a place called 'west'. In contrast, goals are like the places you want to visit while you're travelling west: this bridge, that river, this mountain, that valley; all can be ticked off the list as you go.

So suppose your values in the workplace are to be engaged, efficient, productive, caring and approachable: those values will be there in this job, and the next job and the one after that – whether or not you achieve your goal of finding a dream job. (Of course you may not always act on those values – especially if you don't like your current job – but at any point, should you wish to act on them, you can.)

Here are a few more examples to highlight the difference:

- *To have a big house:* goal. *Caring for and protecting your family:* values.
- *To win the match:* goal. *Playing fairly, enthusiastically and skilfully:* values.
- *To get good marks:* goal. *Applying yourself fully to your studies, and exploring new ideas:* values.
- *To win friends:* goal. *To be warm, friendly, outgoing, supportive and genuine:* values.
- *To lose five kilograms in weight:* goal. *Looking after, strengthening and maintaining your body:* values.
- *To win the race:* goal. *To run to the best of your ability:* value.

Values play a major role in developing confidence and enhancing performance. Not only do they provide us with the inspiration and motivation to 'do what it takes', they also sustain us on the journey; we may be weeks, months or years from completing our goals, but we can live by our values every step of the way, and find ongoing fulfilment in doing so. And even when we *don't* achieve our goals – and at times, we won't – we can still find satisfaction and fulfilment from living by our values.

We'll explore values and goals in more depth later; this is just an appetizer. Now it's time to revisit that important question: what would you do differently if you had more confidence? Take some time to reflect on the answers you gave to the questions on the list on pages 15–16. Hopefully your answers will give you both values and goals. For example, do you want to make more friends, or be more assertive, or become a better conversationalist, or be more focused and engaged, or improve your game of golf, or be a better parent, or expand and develop your business, or increase the openness and intimacy in your marriage, or become more self-accepting, or be more authentic and honest in your relationships, or start that important project, or *complete* that important project, or change careers, or write that book, or pass those exams, or ask that attractive person in your office if they want to go out on a date?

At this point you may not have 'clear' answers. That's absolutely fine. Just come up with some sort of answer, even if it's very vague, or only one word. Later you'll revisit and refine these answers. For now, it's just important to make a start.

Once you've reflected on those questions, write a few words in the following section, 'The Life Change List'. And as you fill it in, see if you can differentiate your values (how you want to behave on an ongoing basis) from your goals (what you want to get, receive, complete or possess). And if you don't want to write in the book, you can either copy the list into your journal, or download a free worksheet at www.thehappinesstrap.co.uk/free_resources.

THE LIFE CHANGE LIST

As I develop genuine confidence . . .

- Here are some ways I will act differently:

- Here are some ways I will treat others differently:

- Here are some ways I will treat myself differently:

- Here are some personal qualities and character strengths I will develop and demonstrate to others:

- Here are some ways I will behave differently in close relationships with friends and family:

- Here are some ways I will behave differently in relationships involving work, education, sport or leisure:

- Here are some important things I will 'stand for':

- Here are some activities I will start or do more of:

- Here are some goals I will work towards:

- Here are some actions I will take to improve my life:

Once you've completed it, please keep your list at hand for ready reference. And please: before reading on, if you haven't actually written anything down, make sure you at least *think seriously* about your answers. (It's okay if they're vague or incomplete, or if you're still unsure of the difference between values and goals; we'll be revisiting all of this later on. All that matters for now is making a start.)

***

So how did you get on? Did you complete the Life Change List, either inside your head or on paper? If so, great; it's an important first step on your path to confidence. If you *haven't* done it, then how about going back and doing it right now? After all, we can't develop karate skills just by reading about them; we have to practise the moves. And it's much the same when it comes to developing confidence. The exercises in this book are all essential moves; if you want to play the confidence game well, you'll need to do them. So please: make sure you have come up with some answers before reading on.

THE CONFIDENCE GAP

Many people are completely lost in something I call the 'confidence gap'. It's that place we get stuck when fear gets in the way of our dreams and ambitions. You know you're stuck in the confidence gap if you believe something like this:

I can't achieve my goals, perform at my peak, do the things I want to do, or behave like the person I want to be, until I feel more confident.

Does this ring true to you? Many self-help approaches inadvertently encourage you to think this way, but you will soon discover that the more tightly you hold on to this belief, the more it will hold you back from creating the life you want. Shortly we'll explore why this is so, but first let's consider the two different definitions of the word 'confidence'.

CONFIDENCE: TWO DEFINITIONS
1.   A feeling of certainty or assurance
2.   An act of trust or reliance

The first definition of confidence – a feeling of certainty or assurance – is by far the most widely used. Most people think of self-confidence as a powerful feeling of certainty or assurance: a sense of being cool, calm and at ease; an absolute belief that you will perform well and achieve a positive outcome; an absence of fear and anxiety; a lack of self-doubt or insecurity; and an absence of negative thoughts about mishaps or failure.

The second definition is used far less commonly. In this definition, confidence is not a *feeling*, but an *action*; it is 'an act of trust or reliance'. This is a much older meaning of the word, which harks back to its ancient origins in Latin. The word 'confidence' is derived from the Latin words 'com', meaning 'with', and 'fidere', meaning 'to trust'. When we trust or rely on someone – whether ourselves or others – we often do *not* have feelings of absolute certainty or assurance. In fact, generally, the more there is at stake, the more we tend to have feelings of fear and anxiety, and thoughts about what might possibly go wrong.

For example, suppose you have a brain tumour and you allow a top neurosurgeon to operate on your brain. That is 'an act of trust or reliance' – you trust or rely on the surgeon to do the operation competently. Another way to say this is that *you have enough confidence* in the surgeon's abilities to let her operate on you. Now it is highly unlikely under these circumstances that you would have feelings of absolute certainty and assurance. Indeed, it would be almost impossible for a human being in this situation to be totally calm and collected, with no fear or anxiety whatsoever. If you're a normal human being facing major brain surgery, you can expect to have plenty of fear and uncertainty, and lots of unpleasant thoughts about the risks.

Both meanings of 'confidence' – a feeling of certainty, or an act of trust – are perfectly valid. But clearly they represent two very different concepts, and we need to distinguish them from one another or we will get confused. So throughout this book, to keep the distinction clear, I will talk about the 'feelings of confidence' or 'confidence, the feeling' as opposed to the 'actions of confidence' or 'confidence, the action'. To see why this distinction is so important, let's consider the story of Nelson Mandela.

'OF COURSE I WAS AFRAID!'

Few individuals have inspired people like Nelson Mandela. He stood for justice, freedom and equality in the face of incredible odds. He risked his life over and over, opposing the brutally oppressive apartheid regime of South Africa, in pursuit of a democratic and free society. It seems a miracle he wasn't killed. But when the South African authorities did eventually capture him, they sentenced him to twenty-seven years in jail, the first eighteen in the atrocious prison on Robben Island.

In his inspiring autobiography, *Long Walk to Freedom*, Mandela describes the horrific conditions in Robben Island prison: slaving all day long under the merciless sun; quarrying and crushing limestone from dawn to dusk; continually subjected to beatings, starvation, and psychological torture. Many men would have crumbled, living year after year in that hell. But not Mandela. He never gave up on his cause. He continued to stand for justice, freedom and equality throughout all those long years of confinement. And against all the odds, he was eventually released from prison, and went on to become the first black president of South Africa.

Richard Stengel, a professional writer who spent two years assisting Mandela with his autobiography, wrote an insightful article in *Time Magazine*, titled 'Mandela: His 8 Lessons of Leadership'. In it, he describes how Mandela frequently felt afraid during his long fight against apartheid and his many years in prison.

'Of course I was afraid!' Mandela told him. 'I can't pretend that I'm brave and that I can beat the whole world.' However, Mandela knew that if he wanted to be a great leader, to inspire his comrades in prison, he had to hide his fear. So that's exactly what he did.

Sure, he couldn't control his feelings, but he had enough control of his facial expressions, his posture and the way he walked and talked to convey the impression of fearlessness to those around him. And this was hugely inspiring to the other prisoners on Robben Island. When they saw him walking through the grounds, holding himself proud and erect, their spirits soared. As Stengel puts it, the sight 'was enough to keep them going for days'.

When Mandela strolled confidently across the prison court-yard, was that an example of 'confidence, the feeling', or 'confidence, the action'? Obviously it was the latter. He was *not* feeling calm, assured and certain. However, he *was* clearly involved in an act of trust. He trusted himself to walk in an 'upright and proud' manner, even though he was feeling very afraid. He did not *eliminate* his fear. He described it as learning to 'triumph over his fear'. In other words, he learned to *rely* on himself; to *trust* himself to take action, no matter how afraid he was feeling.

BACK TO THE GAP

Before our little detours into the different meanings of the word 'confidence' and the prison life of Nelson Mandela, we were talk-ing about 'the confidence gap'. And I said that people get stuck in it when they hold on tightly to this belief: *I have to feel confident before I can achieve my goals, perform at my peak, do the things I want to do, or behave like the person I want to be.*

Now just imagine for a moment that Mandela had played by this rule during his time in prison. Suppose he had waited until all his fear and uncertainty had disappeared *before* he took action. Suppose he had bought into this idea: 'I can't walk across that courtyard holding myself proud and upright until I feel calm, assured and certain; until I have eliminated all my fear; until I have no thoughts about what might go wrong.' Would that have helped him to become an inspirational leader?

Mandela clearly knew how to play the confidence game. He didn't play by the rule: *I have to feel confident before I do what matters.* This is the granddaddy of all those 'wrong rules' I mentioned in the introduction. And the more we play by it, the worse the results.

Now before we go on, I'd like you to pause for ten seconds, and notice what your mind is doing. Just quietly listen in to that voice inside your head, and notice what it is telling you.

***

Is your mind getting annoyed or frustrated: 'Oh please, don't tell me he's going to go down the old "fake it till you make it" path. I've heard that one before!'? Or is it predicting the worst: 'Oh no. He's going to tell me I just have to put up with these feelings of anxiety, grit my teeth, and force myself to do it!'?

If your mind is telling you something like the above, that's perfectly normal and only to be expected; as we shall see later, the human mind has a natural tendency to predict the worst. So let's take this opportunity to clarify something: I am not *ever* going to ask you to 'fake' anything or to 'put up' with unwanted feelings. Quite the opposite, in fact. Two important themes in this book are being true to yourself (as opposed to being 'fake') and handling fear in effective, life-enhancing ways (as opposed to 'putting up with it').

Now, you may be wondering what is so problematic about this rule: *I have to feel confident before I do what matters?* Well, the trouble is, if you wait for the feelings of confidence to show up before you start doing the things that are truly important to you, the chances are you're going to be waiting forever. These feelings are not likely to magically appear out of thin air. Sure, you may be able to cultivate them while you're listening to a self-hypnosis CD, or reading an inspiring book, or participating in a motivational seminar, or when a friend, coach or therapist says something that boosts your confidence. But those feelings don't last. Once you get into the real situation they just vanish in a puff of smoke.

Lance Armstrong, seven-times winner of the Tour de France, and commonly acknowledged as one of the greatest athletes in human history, talks about this subject in his book, *Every Second Counts*. He highlights the fact that vast numbers of people go through life trying to purchase, manufacture or posture self-confidence, and he points out that this is a lost cause. 'You can't fake confidence, you have to earn it', he says. And in his opinion there's only one way to do that: 'You have to do the work.'

This is a key point. If we want to do anything with confidence – speak, paint, make love, play tennis or socialize – then we have to do the work. We have to practise the necessary skills over and over, until they come naturally. If we don't have adequate skills to do the things we want to do, we can't expect to feel confident. And if we don't continually practise these skills, they either get rusty and unreliable, or they never reach a state where we can fluidly and naturally rely on them.

Each time you practise these skills, it is an action of confidence: an act of relying on yourself. And once you have taken action, over and over, so that you have the skills to get the results you want – then you'll start to notice the feelings of confidence.

This insight gives us the first 'right rule' of the confidence game:

Rule 1: The actions *of confidence come first; the* feelings *of confidence come later.*

Of course, it's very easy to say all this, but it's not so easy to do in real life. Why not? Because to develop and practise skills requires time and effort, and our minds usually give us all sorts of reasons not to do it: 'It's too hard', 'I'm too busy', 'I'm not in the mood', 'I've got no motivation', 'I'm too tired', 'I'm too stressed', 'I can't be bothered', 'I'm too anxious', 'I can't do it', 'I've got no discipline', 'There's no point trying because I'll never be any good at it' and so on. When we get caught up in these thoughts, it's all too easy to give up – especially if we're afraid of making mistakes, or we're not feeling too good, or our progress is slower than we'd like.

(By the way, these are perfectly normal thoughts that virtually all human beings have at times, and you're going to learn a new way of responding to them; a way to take all the power out of them, so that no matter how negative the stuff your mind is telling you, you can still take action to do what truly matters to you.)

WHY DO WE LACK CONFIDENCE?

I've never met anyone who lacked confidence in *everything*. I've never even heard of such a person. The fact is, there are many things that we are so incredibly confident at doing, we simply take them for granted. For example, assuming that you are in reasonable health and don't have a significant physical disability, you are probably very confident about walking up and down stairs, using a knife and fork, opening and closing doors, and brushing your teeth. You weren't *always* confident about doing these things; it's just that you've been doing them for so long now, you take them for granted.

So we don't lack confidence in everything; we lack confidence in specific activities, within specific areas of life. And there are five main reasons why this happens.

FIVE REASONS PEOPLE LACK CONFIDENCE

1. Excessive expectations
2. Harsh self-judgement
3. Preoccupation with fear

27

DR RUSS HARRIS

4.   Lack of experience
5.   Lack of skills

Let's quickly go through these.

Excessive expectations
Do you have a mind that is never satisfied? Is it like a little fascist dictator inside your head, always demanding more? If so, you can easily become fearful of making mistakes, and very self-critical if you don't meet your own expectations. This is commonly known as 'perfectionism'. All of us, if we're honest, get caught up in this way of thinking at times. And there's nothing abnormal in that; the human mind is rarely satisfied for long, and is usually quick to find fault and insist on more.

This is the main issue for Dave, the physiotherapist who wants to write a novel. He gets caught up in expectations that every page he writes has to be excellent, even from the very first draft – and because he can't possibly live up to that expectation (no writer can), he doesn't write at all.

Harsh self-judgement
Does your mind undermine you? Does it tell you that you don't have what it takes, or you're no good at what you're doing? Does it say that you're unlikeable, inadequate or incompetent? Does it claim that any moment now you're going to screw it all up? Do you ever suffer from 'impostor syndrome', where your mind manages to convince you that you're not really competent, you don't know what you're doing, you've managed to get away with it so far, but at any moment you will be found out as a fraud? If you answer yes to any of these questions, then that shows you have a *normal* human mind.

Are you surprised to hear that? Most people are, because we've all been brainwashed about positive thinking. But the fact is, the human mind is *not* naturally positive. Eastern models of psychology such as Zen, yoga and the Tao have recognised for thousands of years that the normal human mind has a natural tendency to judge and criticise; to find the negative and predict the worst; to tell us scary stories about the future and dredge up painful memories from the past; to become rapidly dissatisfied and seek more. In the West, we have somehow failed to see that this is the norm; this is what normal minds naturally do. Sadly, most Western models of psychology still believe that when our minds do these things, that's somehow abnormal or unnatural and it means there is something wrong or defective. Fortunately, this attitude is gradually shifting – but it's a slooooow process.

This is the main problem affecting Claire, the attractive but shy receptionist who hasn't dated in four years. She gets so caught up in harsh self-judgements – that she's stupid, unattractive and boring – that she avoids dating, in the belief that men will reject her.

Preoccupation with fear

We all have our own private fears. Perhaps you are fearful of things going wrong or turning out badly. Perhaps you are afraid of rejection, failure or embarrassment. Perhaps you're afraid of making mistakes, wasting your time or making a fool of yourself. Perhaps you are even fearful of fear itself. Such fears are all very common. However, fear in itself does not affect our confidence. But if we dwell on our fears, stew on them and worry about them, that will create problems. The more preoccupied we become with our fears, the greater they grow and the more likely they are to undermine our confidence.

This is the main issue affecting Seb, the taxi driver who avoids making love to his wife. Three years ago he went through a very stressful period when both his parents died in a car crash. During this time, whenever Seb tried to have sex with his wife, he couldn't get an erection, which he found extremely embarrassing. This is completely normal; almost all men find that during times of great stress, they can't obtain erections. But Seb did not know this, and was too embarrassed to discuss it with his friends or his GP. He developed a fear of failure around his sexual performance, worried about it, stewed on it and beat himself up over it. He soon got into a vicious cycle: the more he dwelt on his fear of failure, the worse it became, until eventually he started avoiding sex altogether.

Lack of experience

If we've had little or no experience of doing something, we can't expect to feel confident about it. You might be an excellent guitar player, but if you've never had the experience of playing live before a huge audience, then the first few times you do it, you're highly unlikely to feel confident.

This is Raj's main issue. Raj has plenty of experience at running a successful restaurant, but he's never had the experience of expanding his business and running two restaurants at once; naturally he lacks confidence.

Lack of skill

It's not natural to feel confident about doing something unless we are reasonably good at doing it. For example, I am only just now learning to ride a bicycle, at the age of forty-three. (The kids in my neighbourhood think it is hilarious, watching a grown man wobbling all over the place on his bike.) Now do you think it's realistic for me to feel confident about riding a bike, given I've never previously ridden and I can hardly stay upright? Of course not. If and when, after lots of practice, I become reasonably good at bike-riding, then I may well start to feel confident. But until then, I won't. That's the natural order of things. And it raises an interesting question: how do we become good at doing things?

THE CONFIDENCE CYCLE

If we want to get good at doing anything, we need to follow the four-step Confidence Cycle. You can see this in the diagram below.

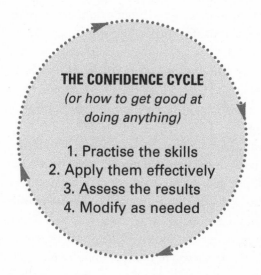

THE CONFIDENCE CYCLE
(or how to get good at doing anything)

1. Practise the skills
2. Apply them effectively
3. Assess the results
4. Modify as needed

Step 1: Practise the skills

If you want to become a confident public speaker, you have to practise giving speeches. If you want to become a confident artist, you have to practise painting. There's no getting away from this fact: if we want to become confident at anything, we have to practise.

The problem is, as we've already noted, there are many mental barriers to practice. These include: lack of motivation or willpower; feeling tired, anxious or fearful; the desire to give up when progress is slow; the tendency to quit after a failure; perfectionism or harsh self-judgement; lack of time, money and energy; and a wide variety of self-limiting beliefs. (As this book progresses, you will learn how to overcome all these mental obstacles.)

Step 2: Apply them effectively

Practising skills is important, but that's not enough to make us good at something. We have also to apply our skills effectively. To apply our skills, we have to step out of our comfort zone and put ourselves into real-life challenging situations. After all, if we repeatedly avoid those situations that challenge us, we'll never be able to test out and improve on our skills. The problem is, leaving our comfort zone brings up all sorts of discomfort – such as fear, anxiety or self-doubt. Fortunately, mindfulness helps us transcend these feelings.

Furthermore, if we want to act effectively in challenging situations, we need to be able to focus on what we are doing. Psychologists call this 'task-focused attention'. If we get all caught up in our thoughts and feelings, we won't be able to focus on what we are doing, and therefore we won't do it very well. The mindfulness skills you'll learn in this book will help you to stay engaged and absorbed in whatever you're doing, from playing football to playing the trumpet, from making love to making a sales pitch. And this will not only improve your performance, but also increase your sense of fulfilment.

Step 3: Assess the results

After we apply our skills, we need to reflect on the results. What did we do that worked? What did we do that didn't work? How could we do it differently next time around? And we need to do this non-judgementally – without beating ourselves up.

Now, this is usually easier said than done. Most of us have a strong perfectionist streak – we want to get it right and do it well.

And our minds have a tendency to pull out the whip and give us a good lashing if we don't measure up to our own expectations. Unfortunately, harsh self-judgement is always unproductive. It rarely spurs us on to greater things but just makes us feel like giving up. So later in the book, you'll learn how mindfulness can help you to circumvent this. And you'll discover that non-judgemental self-reflection and compassionate self-encouragement will be far more helpful than beating yourself up.

Step 4: Modify as needed
The final step, based upon the results you get, is to modify what you are doing. You do more of what is working well, and you change or modify what is not working so well. This is the only way to develop and improve. As the saying goes, 'If you do what you've always done, you'll get what you've always gotten.'

And then of course you repeat the cycle. You practise your skills with the new modifications, then you apply them again, assess the results and modify them further; and then you practise some more, and so on. And then, eventually, you will be good at doing it. And if your mind is saying this all seems like too much hard work, then consider this:

YOU HAVE DONE THIS MANY TIMES BEFORE!
Just for a moment, think about all the things you can confidently do today; things you do so fluidly and naturally, you rarely even stop to consider them. For example, you can use a knife and fork to eat, a pen to write, and a kettle to boil water. You can walk, talk, read books, go shopping, make toast, open a can, use a toilet, run a bath, tell the time, recite the alphabet and dress yourself . . . all with the greatest of ease. And how did you learn to do this?

You had to practise, practise, practise all these skills, continually assessing the results and modifying what you'd done. Through that process you developed these skills to such an extent that you can now do them naturally, fluidly and confidently. (And if your mind's protesting that some people have 'natural ability', of course that's true; but they still have to run through the above cycle many, many times to get good at something. All 'natural ability' means is that they don't have to work as hard as the rest of us to reach the same level of skill.)

THE USUAL SUSPECTS

So whenever we lack self-confidence, the usual suspects are: excessive expectations, harsh self-judgement, preoccupation with fear, lack of experience, and lack of skill. And we're going to address all of these issues in time. For now, let's just acknowledge one more time that developing genuine confidence requires work. Or rather, it requires 'committed action'.

In ACT, we use the term 'committed action' to mean action that we take guided by our core values: behaving like the person we want to be, and doing what truly matters to us. Only through committed action – stepping out of our comfort zones and doing what truly matters deep in our hearts – will we experience authentic confidence.

Now take a moment to notice what you are thinking. For twenty seconds, stop reading, close your eyes and simply notice what your mind is saying.

***

I'm hoping your mind will be all 'fired up' and eager to go, but you may find that it is groaning or complaining, or protesting that this all sounds too hard, or predicting that it won't work for you and telling you to give up. All of these different reactions are normal and natural, so whatever your mind is saying – whether it's being positive or negative, encouraging or discouraging, enthusiastic or doubtful – just notice it without trying to change it.

Now, as we're fast approaching the end of the chapter, let's quickly summarise the key points:

KEY POINTS

- Consider what you would do if you had more confidence, and write a Life Change List
- Remember rule #1 of the confidence game: *The actions of confidence come first; the feelings of confidence come later*
- Identify the main causes of your low self-confidence: excessive expectations, harsh self-judgement, preoccupation with fear, lack of experience or lack of skill
- Remember the Confidence Cycle: practise the skills, apply them effectively, assess the results and modify as needed

DOES 'INSTANT CONFIDENCE' REALLY EXIST?

There are many books, courses and seminars that claim they can provide you with 'instant confidence'. And 'instant confidence' is a very good name for what they offer – because it only lasts for an instant. What typically happens is that for a brief instant – while we are reading the book in the safety of our bedrooms, or listening to that CD in our cars, or participating in the buzz and drama of a seminar – we can conjure up those feelings of confidence. But as soon as we get into a real situation, stepping out of our comfort zones, facing a genuine challenge in real life – then all those wonderful feelings just evaporate. Poof! Gone! Vanished! And there's a very good reason for why this happens. To understand it, we need to go back in time to . . .

chapter 2

the good old days

It's coming for you!

Thump! Thump! Thump!

The ground beneath your feet is trembling.

Thump! Thump! Thump!

The beast raises its mighty trunk into the air and lets out a blood-curdling bellow. It's three times your height, covered with shaggy brown hair, has legs the size of tree trunks, and two enormous tusks protruding from its mouth.

It's angry. And it's running at you!

Thump! Thump! Thump!

So what happens next? You'll find out shortly. First let's backtrack to the granddaddy of all those 'wrong rules' for the confidence game: *I have to feel confident before I do what matters.* This rule appeals to 'common sense' because it's often much easier to take action and do the things that are important to you if you're already feeling confident. But clinging tightly to this belief means you will spend a lot of time, effort and energy trying to control your feelings. And you will probably try very hard to eliminate feelings of fear, anxiety and uncertainty, and replace them with those of calm, certainty and assurance. Indeed, plenty of popular self-help books claim to show you just how to do that, via positive affirmations, challenging negative thoughts, self-hypnosis and so on. Unfortunately, it's just not that easy to control your feelings, and the further you go down that road, the more likely you are to feel disappointed, frustrated or hopeless.

But please don't take my word for it; check your own experience. Have you ever found a technique for controlling your feelings (without using powerful drugs) that works when you are in a truly challenging situation, stepping out of your comfort zone and facing your fears? Have you found a technique that enables you to feel total certainty and assurance under those conditions? This question is a set-up. I know you haven't, because it's impossible; there's no way to undo billions of years of evolution that have hardwired your body to respond to such challenging situations in a very specific manner: with something called the 'fight-or-flight response'.

To explain what this is, let's return to that mammoth. When a woolly mammoth is charging straight towards you, you really only have two options. Option one: run away (very, very, very, very fast!). Option two: stay your ground and fight (very, very, very, very hard!). Really, that's about it: fight or flight. And note that both responses require lots of energy. In order to fight or take flight you need power, strength and stamina. (Otherwise, you get squashed.)

Fortunately, thanks to hundreds of millions of years of evolution, your body will provide you with exactly what you need. When you face a threat, your body floods with adrenaline, your reflexes become faster, your muscles tense for action, your focus sharpens, and your heart pumps extra blood to the parts of your body that need it most – primarily the large muscles of your arms and legs. We call this amazing reaction the 'fight-or-flight' response. (Technically speaking, it's the 'fight, flight or freeze' response, because sometimes we 'freeze' instead of fleeing or fighting – but for the sake of simplicity we'll stick to the shorter version.)

All mammals, as well as fish, reptiles and birds, have a fight-or-flight response. It is immediate and automatic. Essential for survival, it activates the moment an animal perceives a threat. It prepares you to fight off the threat, or take flight from it – whichever is most likely to save your life. Suppose your primitive ancestor, facing that charging woolly mammoth, did *not* have such a response. Suppose they just stood there, watching and waiting, marvelling at the beauty and majesty of the charging behemoth. They soon would have been very flat!

Now, let's imagine you're part of a group of our cave-dwelling ancestors, living together in a happy little prehistoric valley. And let's suppose that life is good in that valley. You know where the food is, you know where the water is, you know who your neighbours are – and you know where the dangerous animals are, so you can keep well away from them. But you also know full well that you can't stay in your happy little valley all the time; every so often, you'll need to go out looking for food. Whenever the food supplies run low, you get together with your neighbours and set off over the mountain to see if you can bag a woolly mammoth for dinner.

But this is no small undertaking. You're taking a significant risk. The further you travel from your old familiar territory, the more danger you're in. After all, there are big animals out there. With big claws and big teeth. Animals that would love nothing more than to have a puny hairless ape for a lunchtime snack! So you need to be on the lookout: alert for sabre-toothed tigers, hungry cave-bears and rival clans.

At the slightest hint of a threat – a sudden movement in the bushes, an odd smell in the air, a strange shadow on the horizon – your fight-or-flight response kicks in. Your heart races, you flood with adrenaline, your muscles tense. This is a good thing; now you are ready to fight or take flight. And if it turns out to be a false alarm, no problem: after a while, in the absence of any threat, the response will cease. Your adrenaline levels will come down, your heart rate will drop, and you'll feel more relaxed.

Things haven't changed all that much since those ancestral days. Sure, life is a bit easier, and there's much less risk of being eaten, gored or stomped on by big animals, but we still have to take risks. If we want to grow and develop as human beings, we have to step out of our old familiar territory and venture into the unknown. And we will have to do this not just once, but again and again. And each time we leave that familiar territory – popularly known as the 'comfort zone' – our fight-or-flight response will be triggered.

Now, this is completely natural. Each time you leave your comfort zone to enter a challenging new situation, you are taking a significant risk. After all, there's no assurance that things will turn out the way you want. The inconvenient truth is that bad things *can* happen. No one can guarantee that they won't. You might fail, or get hurt, or screw it up, or make a fool of yourself. You might be rejected, or lose all your money, or waste time and effort, ending up with nothing to show for it. And the greater the step you take outside of your comfort zone – the greater the challenge you face – the more uncertainty there is about the outcome. Under these circumstances, there is no way that you will be able to 'switch off' your fight-or-flight response; no way to instil yourself with feelings of absolute certainty and assurance. (That is, apart from using drugs with dangerous side effects.)

Of course, in everyday language, we don't usually talk about the fight-or-flight response. You've probably never heard someone say, 'I'm giving a talk in front of two hundred people next week and I'm having a fight-or-flight response.' You're far more likely to hear talk of fear or nervousness.

WHAT'S IN A NAME?

Fear has many different names. Here are a few of the more common ones: 'lack of confidence', 'anxiety', 'self-doubt', 'insecurity', 'nerves', 'cold feet', 'stressing out'. I've worked with CEOs, soldiers, police officers, lawyers and surgeons who initially refused to admit to having 'fear' or 'anxiety', because they saw these emotions as a personal failing, or a sign of weakness. They *could* admit to being 'stressed', 'tense', 'wired' or having 'a crisis of confidence', but not to being 'anxious' or 'afraid'.

This is hardly surprising. In almost every human culture, fear is demonized as a sign of personal weakness – especially in men. And in our society, the brainwashing starts very young. Think about it. When you were a little kid and you were feeling frightened, what kinds of unhelpful things did adults say to you? And in the process, what messages did they send you about fear?

For example, did you ever hear 'Don't be silly; there's nothing to be afraid of,' or 'Don't be stupid. There's no such thing as ghosts (or monsters, or vampires)'? The message here is: feeling afraid means being silly or stupid. Maybe you heard some of these: 'Don't be such a baby', 'Grow up' or 'Act your age.' And suppose you were so scared you actually started to cry; then you may have heard: 'Don't be a cry-baby', 'Don't be a cissy', 'Big boys don't cry.' The message here is that fear equals immaturity or weakness.

And these messages are powerfully reinforced by pop culture. In virtually every book, comic, movie or TV series, the heroes and heroines are . . . *fearless*. Indiana Jones, Charlie's Angels, James

Bond, Wonder Woman, Superman, Batman: they have no fear! Okay, occasionally, just occasionally, they do reveal a tiny glimpse of it. For example, I do remember one James Bond movie where you actually saw a few droplets of sweat on his forehead. The film was *Dr No*, and the scene I'm thinking of had Sean Connery strapped to a table, legs akimbo, and a laser beam was about to slice his testicles off. So in that situation, he was allowed to have a bit of sweat on his forehead. But when the whole world is about to blow up, all he does is smile and crack a joke.

With all of this conditioning going on, it's hardly surprising we grow up with a negative attitude towards fear. This is a great shame, because as we'll see later in the book, fear is like a powerful fuel; once we know how to handle it, we can use it to our advantage; we can harness its energy to help us get where we want. But while we're looking at fear as something 'bad', we'll waste a lot of precious energy trying to avoid or get rid of it.

Now, once again, pause for a moment and for ten seconds, notice what your mind is telling you.

***

So, is your mind on board for the ride, eager to find out more? Or is it saying, 'This guy's full of it. Clearly I bought the wrong book. This isn't what I wanted to hear'?

Whatever your mind is saying is fine by me. I fully expect that as you keep reading, there will be times when your mind is very enthusiastic, and other times it will be very sceptical and critical. That's just what minds do. So see if you can let your mind chatter away – like a voice on a radio playing in the background – and carry on working through the book. And see if you can stay open to the reality that you will *not* develop true confidence – in either sense of the word – by trying to eliminate fear, 'nerves' or anxiety.

However, you *will* develop true confidence, in both senses of the word, once you learn how to change your relationship with fear and use it to your advantage. But before we get to that point, there's a little more myth-busting to be done. And what better way to start than with a game of . . .

chapter 3

true or false?

Ready for a little quiz? Please answer true or false to each statement:

1. Albert Einstein was a below-average school student.
2. You only use 10 per cent of your brain.
3. Positive self-statements, such as 'I will succeed' or 'I am lovable', are a good way to boost low self-esteem.

Most people answer 'true' for most or all of these statements. This is only to be expected. After all, countless books, TV programmes and articles on self-improvement tell you these things as if they were hard facts. They tell you Einstein did poorly at school. (The message: if Einstein could go on to such greatness despite his early failures, then so can you.) They tell you that you use just ten per cent of your brain. (The message: imagine what you could achieve if you used all of your brain.) They tell you positive self-statements will give you high self-esteem. (The message: it's easy to eliminate negative self-talk.)

As you may have guessed from my tone, all these widely known, frequently quoted 'facts' are actually false. Yes, Einstein did do poorly in French in his early teen years, but overall he was a good student, excelling in maths and physics, and his marks in all subjects averaged more than 80 per cent in his final year at school. As for only using 10 per cent of your brain – hmm. This idea started in the early 1900s, but has been popularized in the past fifty years. Yet despite the fact that thousands of self-development programmes quote this 'fact', you will never see one shred of hard scientific evidence to support it. And that is because it is complete and utter nonsense. Scientists have studied the brain extensively in a myriad of different ways – from MRI and PET scans to examination under a microscope. And guess what? They have never located one single part of the brain that is redundant. Every part of it serves a function, and you use 100 per cent of it every day. If a stroke, tumour, disease or injury destroys even a tiny percentage of the brain, this usually results in significant disability.

And what about positive affirmations? Chances are you've read or been told that if you're experiencing self-doubt, or low self-esteem, or generally lacking confidence in yourself, then the solution is to think positive things about yourself, over and over, until you believe them. Have you ever tried doing this? If so, did it work for you? Or did you find that it just caused your mind to get into an argument with itself?

While motivational speakers and self-help gurus love to espouse the benefits of positive affirmations – and the concept certainly appeals to 'common sense' – there is no scientific evidence to show it works. In fact, science suggests the very opposite!

In 2009, a team of Canadian psychologists – Joanne V. Wood and John W. Lee from the University of Waterloo, and W Q Elaine Perunovic from the University of New Brunswick – published a groundbreaking study in *Psychological Science* magazine (which is ranked among the top ten psychology journals in the world). Their study, entitled 'Positive Self-Statements: Power for some, peril for others', made world headlines. Why? Because it showed that people with low self-esteem actually feel *worse* after repeating positive self-statements such as 'I am a lovable person' or 'I will succeed.'

Rather than being helpful, these positive thoughts typically triggered a strong negative reaction and a resultant low mood. For example, if a participant with low self-esteem said to herself, 'I am a lovable person', her mind would answer back, 'No you're not!' and run through a list of all the ways in which she was *not* lovable. Not surprisingly, this would make her feel even worse than before. On the other hand, when these participants were told it was okay to have negative thoughts about themselves, their moods lifted!

So what's all this got to do with confidence? Well, the connection is a bit oblique, but it does demonstrate the fact that . . .

WE'RE ALL FULL OF IT!

Hopefully you're starting to see that we all walk around with our heads full of inaccurate and misleading information. (Confession: I, too, once believed all the above myths.) We are all too ready to believe all sorts of seemingly 'common sense' ideas without stopping to question their origin or validity. And this is especially so in the realm of pop psychology. It's important to keep this in mind, because if we hold on tightly to these ideas, they can create all sorts of problems for us. As the great writer Mark Twain put it: 'It ain't what you don't know that gets you into trouble. It's what you know for sure that just ain't so.' So with this in mind, let's quickly review four widely held beliefs: fear is a sign of weakness; fear impairs performance; fear holds you back; and confidence is the absence of fear.

Myth: Fear is a sign of weakness

Do you buy into this idea? Then let me quote you a couple of people whom you could hardly call 'weak': legendary long-distance cyclist Lance Armstrong, one of the greatest athletes of all time; and blockbuster movie star Hugh Jackman, whose rippling muscles cause both men and women to swoon.

'I fear failure. I have a huge phobia around failure.' Lance Armstrong

'I've always felt that if you back down from a fear, the ghost of that fear never goes away. It diminishes people. So I've always said "yes" to the thing I'm most scared about.' Hugh Jackman

Now stop reading, and for a few seconds notice what your mind is telling you.

***

So did you hear your mind protest with something like this, 'Yes, but it's different for them. I'm not competing in the Tour de France, or starring in Hollywood movies, so I *shouldn't* be afraid.'

If your mind did tell you something like that, it's hardly surprising. It takes time to fully assimilate the information we discussed in the previous chapter about the fight–or–flight response. The fact is, every normal human being experiences this response when they step out of their comfort zone into a challenging situation. This is not a sign of weakness, but a sign of normality. If you don't experience this response when you take a risk, face a challenge, or leave your comfort zone it means one of two things: a) there's something seriously wrong with your brain; or b) you're a fictitious character like James Bond.

46

Now, the size and shape of your comfort zone is inevitably going to be different to that of Armstrong or Jackman – or your parents or your children or your next-door-neighbour's mother-in-law. That's a given; we're all individuals. But no matter how big or small your comfort zone is, the fact is, the moment you leave it you're going to have a fight-or-flight response. And the greater the step you take, the stronger the response, and the greater the fear you'll experience. At the risk of repeating myself:

When you step out of your comfort zone, take a risk, or face a challenge you will feel fear. That's not weakness; it's the natural state of affairs for normal human beings.

Now, as you work through this book, I expect your comfort zone to expand. And as this happens, where you once struggled with fear, anxiety and self-doubt you are likely to be much more at ease and able to engage fully in what you are doing, without an ongoing battle with your thoughts and feelings. But there's no way to expand your comfort zone without stepping out of it – and the moment you take that step, fear is going to show up.

Myth: Fear impairs performance

Talk to a few top athletes, movie stars, public speakers, musicians or other stage performers and you'll soon discover this is not true. When performers put themselves out there in the public arena, the indisputable fact is that they are taking a risk. No matter how accomplished they are, no matter how much their fans love them, no matter how successful they've been in the past, there's always the chance that this time they could screw it up. The fact is, they face a genuinely challenging situation that taxes their skills and abilities. And when any human being takes a risk and faces a genuinely challenging situation, what do they experience? That's right: a fight-or-flight response.

However, top performers rarely refer to this response as 'fear', 'anxiety' or 'nerves'. They are more likely to call it being pumped, revved up or amped, or having an adrenaline rush. When people use words such as these, rather than words like 'fear' or 'anxiety', then they have discovered this very important truth:

Fear is not your enemy. It is a powerful source of energy that can be harnessed and used for your benefit.

Most top performers instinctively know this; they learn how to channel their fear and anxiety into their performance – and in doing so, the quality of their performance increases. This may sound hard to believe, but later in the book, you'll learn how to do this yourself.

Myth: Fear holds you back

This is really a variant of the last two myths. The story is that fear somehow holds you back from achieving what you want in life. Luckily, this isn't the case. What holds you back is not fear, but your attitude towards it. The tighter you hold on to the attitude that fear is something 'bad' and you can't do the things you want until it goes away, the more stuck you will be. In fact, that very attitude – that fear is something 'bad' – will not only keep you stuck, but it will actually increase your fear; it leads to fear about your fear, anxiety about your anxiety, nerves about your nerves. (Indeed, this attitude plays a major role in all common anxiety disorders, from panic disorder to social phobia.)

I mentioned earlier that top performers learn to accept their fear and channel it into their performance. However, occasionally a performer buys into the idea that fear is 'bad' – and the moment they adopt that attitude, they develop 'stage fright'. All of a sudden, their fear becomes a serious problem, a major obstacle, something they struggle with. And generally the more they struggle with it, the worse it gets. The simple fact is this:

It is not fear that holds people back – it is their attitude towards it that keeps them stuck.

Some performers struggle with their fear so much that they even start taking drugs or cancelling their performances – or both – hoping to make it go away. But this is futile. To quote Eleanor Roosevelt: 'You gain strength, courage and confidence by every experience in which you really stop to look fear in the face. The danger lies in refusing to face the fear, in not daring to come to grips with it.'

Myth: Confidence is the absence of fear

The story goes that confident people don't feel anxious or afraid. This is simply not so. Refer back to the first two myths. The fact is, in a challenging situation, even the most confident people on the planet experience fear. However, when you know how to handle it effectively, it does not destroy your confidence. This gives us the second rule of the confidence game:

Rule 2: Genuine confidence is not the absence of fear; it is a transformed relationship *with fear.*

IN SUMMARY

In the next section of the book, we're going to knuckle down to the real work: learning and practising the skills that will enable you to transform your relationship with fear and develop genuine confidence. But before we finish, here's a quick recap of the main points in this chapter:

KEY POINTS
- When you step out of your comfort zone, take a risk or face a challenge, you will feel fear. That's not weakness; it's the normal state of affairs for normal human beings
- Fear is not your enemy. It is a powerful source of energy that can be harnessed and used for your benefit
- It is not fear that holds people back – it is their attitude towards fear that keeps them stuck
- Genuine confidence is not the absence of fear; it is a transformed relationship with fear

So, are you ready to fundamentally transform your relationship with fear; to stop regarding it as an enemy and turn it into a powerful source of energy? If so, the first step is learning how to handle that double-edged sword, the mind.

part two

the double-edged sword

chapter 4

it ain't necessarily so

What's it like for you?

Is it like a voice inside your head: 'You'll fail', 'You don't have what it takes', 'You'll get rejected', 'You'll screw it up', 'It could all go horribly wrong' or 'You're not ready for it yet – better put it off until later'? Or is it more like a sensation in your body: churning stomach, clenched teeth, tight throat, pounding heart, restless legs, tense muscles, tight chest, difficulty breathing, dry mouth and/or sweaty hands?

Whatever you prefer to call it – lack of confidence, fear of failure, anxiety, nerves or tension – it boils down to a few basic elements, which are described by psychologists as 'private experiences', because they are experiences that only you know about. The most common private experiences that the human brain and nervous system EMITS are these:

E – Emotions
M – Memories

I – Images
T – Thoughts
S – Sensations

So usually, when someone talks about a 'lack of self-confidence', they are referring to some of the following:

- Emotions such as fear and anxiety
- Memories of past failures or mistakes
- Images (ie mental pictures) of things going badly
- Thoughts about failure, disaster, doing it wrong, not being good enough or giving up, and
- Sensations such as a racing heart, dry mouth or butter-flies in the stomach.

In this book, for the sake of simplicity, I am going to lump all these 'private experiences' into two categories. Memories, thoughts and images I will simply refer to as 'thoughts'. Emotions and sensations I will call 'feelings'. And when I use the term 'thoughts and feel-ings', I mean every private experience a human has: emotions, memories, images, thoughts and sensations.

Now, to develop lasting confidence, we need to know three things:

- How to handle our thoughts and feelings effectively
- How to take control of our actions, even when our thoughts and feelings are 'negative' or uncomfortable
- How to engage fully in whatever we are doing, irre-spective of the thoughts and feelings we are having

I'm going to leave feelings until later in the book, because they're easier to deal with once we can handle our thoughts. So let's begin by considering . . .

WHAT ARE THOUGHTS?

Thoughts are words and pictures inside our head. (Psychologists' technical term for 'thought' is 'cognition'.) There are many different categories of thoughts, including memories, images, fantasies, beliefs, ideas, attitudes, assumptions, values, goals, plans, visions, dreams, desires, predictions, judgements and so on. But no matter how complex our thoughts may be, they are all constructed from two basic building blocks: words and images.

Check this out for yourself: when you get to the row of asterisks below, stop reading for one minute, close your eyes, and simply notice what your mind is doing. You should notice either some words – which you 'hear' like a voice or 'see' like writing – or some pictures, or a combination of both. (If your mind goes blank, just wait; it won't take long before your mind says something like 'I'm not having any thoughts' – which is, of course, a thought.) Please try this now for one minute.

***

So what did you notice? What did your mind have to say to or show you? (If you noticed sensations or feelings in your body as opposed to words and pictures in your head, I would not call those 'thoughts', I'd call them 'sensations' or 'feelings'; we'll deal with them later.) You've undoubtedly noticed that your mind is very good at generating words and pictures. Consider for a moment: how many thoughts does your mind create in the space of just one day? Hundreds upon thousands, if not millions. And it never runs out, does it? It's always 'show and tell' time for the mind; it's always got something to say, or something to show us.

And you've undoubtedly also noticed that your mind has a tendency to be negative. As I said in chapter 1, that's perfectly natural and normal. The human mind is quick to judge, criticize, compare, point out what's not good enough, and tell us what needs to be improved. And although our culture bombards us with messages about the importance of positive thinking, the simple fact is this: *the human mind has evolved to think negatively.*

To understand why this is, let's return to our primitive ancestors. Most scientists agree that our species, *Homo sapiens*, appeared around 100,000 years ago. In those days, we had four basic needs: food, water, shelter and sex. (Not all at the same time, mind you – gets a bit messy.) But none of these things is important if you're dead. So back then the number one job that your mind had to do – better than any other job – was to stop you getting killed.

So how does a mind do that?

It looks around for danger. It constantly scans the environment, trying to spot or anticipate anything that can possibly hurt you.

A hundred thousand years ago, if your mind was not very good at doing this job, then you didn't live very long! Bears, wolves, sabre-toothed tigers, woolly mammoths, avalanches, volcanos, rival tribes and jealous neighbours: there was no shortage of painful or violent ways to die. So if there ever was an early human who went through life in a fearless and carefree manner, only noticing all the good things around them, thinking positively that nothing would ever go wrong, they would have been eaten, trampled or murdered pretty quickly – long before they had a chance to reproduce!

You and I evolved from the cavemen and cavewomen who were always on the lookout: always alert for danger; always prepared for the worst. So our modern brains are always trying to anticipate what could hurt us or harm us; always trying to predict what might go wrong. No wonder we all have so many doubts, worries, concerns and fears of failure. This is not a sign of a weak or defective mind; it's a perfectly natural by-product of evolution. And that is why, even if we diligently practise positive thinking every single day of our lives, *we can't stop our minds from generating negative thoughts!*

Many people are surprised to hear this. After all, our society bombards us with messages about the importance of positive thinking. (There is even a popular brand of bottled water that says on the label, 'Drink Positive, Think Positive!' Please – give us a break. Can't we even drink some water in peace, without being hassled about how we think?) Unfortunately, what these books, articles and courses on positive thinking often fail to mention is that although we can learn to think a bit more positively, that won't stop negative thoughts from arising.

Anything you've read in self-help books about 'erasing old mental tapes' or 'deleting old programmes' or 'eliminating negative core beliefs' is stuff and nonsense. The latest discoveries in the world of neuroscience make it very clear that the brain does not eliminate or eradicate old neural pathways; rather it lays down new ones *on top* of the old ones. The more you use these new neural pathways, the more habitual your new patterns of thinking will become. But those old neural pathways will not disappear; those old patterns of thinking will not vanish.

It's a bit like cutting a new path through a forest. The more the new pathway is used, the more established it becomes. But the old path doesn't cease to exist. If it gets used less often, the grass may grow over it to some degree, but it's still there – and easily 'reclaimed'. The problem with this analogy is that it is easy to stop using an old pathway in a forest; it's a billion times harder to stop using an old pathway in your brain.

So here's another analogy that might be better. When you practise new types of thinking, it's like learning to speak a new language. But no matter how fluent you become in the new language, your old language doesn't disappear. No matter how well you learn to speak Spanish, you won't lose the ability to speak English.

THE GREATEST ZEN MASTER IN THE LAND

When it comes to training the mind to perform at its peak, Zen masters are the equivalent of Olympic athletes. So it's worth heeding this ancient Zen parable. One day in the monastery, a novice approaches the head monk and says, 'Master, how do I find the greatest Zen master in the whole land?'

The head monk scratches his head, and thinks for a moment. Then he says, 'Find the man who tells you he has eliminated all negative thoughts. And if you find such a man, you'll know that's *not* who you're looking for.'

In other words, even the greatest Zen masters have negative thoughts. And so do the greatest 'positive psychologists'. The world-famous psychologist Martin Seligman provides a good example. Seligman, the author of hugely successful books such as *Learned Optimism* and *Authentic Happiness,* is widely referred to as 'the father of positive psychology'. And one of the many things I admire about Seligman is his honesty: he admits that even though he has spent the last twenty years teaching people all around the world to think optimistically, as soon as he finds himself in a challenging situation, the first thing that pops into his head is a pessimistic thought. Now just stop reading for twenty seconds, and notice what your mind is telling you.

***

Is your mind protesting, arguing or criticizing? Or is it relieved to know that you're normal? Is it perhaps excited and curious about what comes next? Or is it worried that I'm going to tell you that this is your lot in life and you have to just put up with it? Please let your mind say whatever it wants; you'll have noticed it's always got an opinion! Of course, at times those opinions are useful. But at other times, they're extremely unhelpful. Which is why, in ACT, we say . . .

THE MIND IS A DOUBLE-EDGED SWORD

Our minds are pretty amazing. They help us plan for the future and learn from the past. They help us analyse our world and generate useful guidelines for living and thriving. They enable us to communicate, negotiate and contribute; to innovate, improve and invent; to be creative and adaptive.

That's the bright side.

The dark side of the mind is that it's quick to criticize and judge harshly. It conjures up scary stories about the future, and dredges up painful memories from the past. It reminds us of our flaws, faults and failures, and compares us unfavourably to others. And there is nothing abnormal or defective about any of this; these are all the ordinary processes of a normal human mind.

Later in the book we'll look at how to use the 'bright side' of the mind: how to clarify our values, set goals and think strategically, to help us with motivation and commitment. But in this section, we're going to focus on the 'dark side'; on handling all those inevitable negative thoughts. And if you're wondering, 'Are they *really* inevitable?' – well, let's see.

THE 'POP-UP THOUGHTS' EXERCISE

Here's a little exercise invented by Steven Hayes. I'm about to give you three well-known phrases – but in each case, the last word is missing. As you read the incomplete sentences, notice what words automatically pop into your head. This is not a quiz – I don't want you to guess the answers – I want you to simply notice what pops into your head without any effort at all. Here goes:

- Children should be seen and not . . .

- Mary had a little ...
- Blondes have more ...

So what happened? If you grew up in the UK, Australia, the US, Canada or New Zealand, speaking English as your first language, then the words that probably popped into your head were: 'heard', 'lamb' and 'fun'. So, do you really believe that children should be seen and not heard? Or that there really was a girl called Mary who had a little lamb that followed her to school? Or that blondes really do have more fun than people of other hair colours? I'm betting the answer in each case is no. So now suppose I said to you: eliminate all of those word sequences from your mind; eradicate them so that under no circumstances do those specific sequences of words ever pop up again inside your head. Could you do that? Maybe with science-fiction brain surgery – but otherwise they are deeply implanted in your mind. We can pretty much guarantee that in a context where someone says, 'Mary had a little . . .', the word 'lamb' will pop up inside your head. And your mind is full of this stuff. Let's try a few more: read these sentences and notice the words your brain supplies automatically.

- Every cloud has a ...
- Diamonds are a girl's ...
- Plenty more fish in ...
- You only use 10 per cent of ...

***

Just as the word 'lamb' pops up when we encounter the phrase 'Mary had a little', negative thoughts will pop up whenever we encounter a genuinely challenging situation. Like it or not, as soon as we even *think* about stepping out of our comfort zones, our minds are likely to tell us those same old stories; the ones they've been telling us ever since we were young. You know the ones I mean: 'You'll fail', or 'You'll screw it up', or 'It'll go wrong', or 'You're not ready', or 'You're not good enough', or 'It's too hard' and so on. We can bundle all these thoughts up into one big story: 'I can't do it'.

In chapter 1 I mentioned Claire, the somewhat shy thirty-three-year-old receptionist who hasn't been out on a date in more than four years. Her version of the 'I can't do it' story was: 'I can't start dating, because I don't know how to talk to guys; I get so nervous, I just clam up.' I also mentioned Raj, the successful businessman who wanted to open up a second restaurant. His version of the story was, 'I can't do it because I might fail and lose a lot of money.' Then there was Dave, the physiotherapist who dreamed of writing novels. His story was short and sweet: 'I can't write!' There was also Alexis, the mother of two who wanted to stand up to her domineering, hypercritical mother-in-law. Alexis's version went: 'I can't do it because it's too scary. I don't know how she'll react.' And for one last example, let's revisit Seb, the taxi driver who avoided making love to his wife; his version of the story was 'I can't do it because it's too embarrassing; I'm too scared it might happen again.'

Over the past five years, I have spoken on this topic to thousands of people in Australia, UK, the US and Europe, to widely varying audiences including doctors, lawyers, police officers, business executives, CEOs, psychologists, counsellors, therapists, coaches, psychiatrists, athletes, entrepreneurs and parents' groups, and I always ask this question: 'Is there anyone in this room who can honestly put their hand up and say that they do *not* have some version of the "I can't do it" story?' So far, not one single person has ever raised their hand.

So if you can't stop your mind from telling you the 'I can't do it' story, then what are you supposed to do when this story shows up? The three most common solutions you'll encounter are a) challenge or dispute the thoughts, and look for evidence to prove they're not true; b) replace them with more positive thoughts; c) distract yourself from the thoughts.

Now, you may like to try these things out if you've never done so before. However, given that these solutions are the ones that almost everyone will suggest to you, I expect you've already tried them. And if you *have* tried them, you've undoubtedly recognised that a) they require a lot of effort and energy: b) even if they do give you temporary relief from negative thoughts, your mind just keeps on coming up with new ones: and c) when you leave your comfort zone to enter a genuinely challenging situation, these techniques don't help you very much. (You may even have found, as in the research I mentioned before, that trying to think positively made you feel worse.)

SO WHAT'S THE ALTERNATIVE?

If you're familiar with ACT, you know what's coming. But if you're not, you're probably wondering: 'So what am I supposed to do then? Am I just supposed to ignore these thoughts? Or grit my teeth and put up with them? Or try to push them away? Or try to distract myself from them?'

Personally, I wouldn't recommend any of these strategies. Again, I'm willing to bet you've already tried doing these things – they are commonsense approaches that almost everyone tries at some point. And if you have, you probably found that even if they gave you some short-term benefits, they didn't, in the long run, give you an empowering and life-enhancing way of dealing effectively with negative thoughts.

Therefore, you're going to learn a radically different way of responding to negative thoughts; something that will go against almost everything you have been taught growing up in our society. But first let's consider a very important question.

ARE NEGATIVE THOUGHTS REALLY A PROBLEM?

How many times have you heard or read (or perhaps even told someone else) that negative thoughts are bad, problematic, harmful or self-defeating? That you 'shouldn't be thinking that way'? That 'winners' think positively, and 'losers' think negatively? That negative thinking will hold you back? That happy people don't have those kinds of thoughts? That thinking that way will give you poor self-esteem, or low self-confidence?

Chances are, people have been engraving these ideas into your brain ever since you were a toddler. You've heard them over and over from parents, teachers, self-help books, friends, health professionals, TV programmes, newspapers and magazines. The most extreme version takes the line that your negative thoughts are so harmful that they will actually manifest in reality; they will actually come true. Hmm. Interesting proposition; let's look at it a bit more closely.

You may be familiar with a common anxiety disorder called OCD (obsessive-compulsive disorder). Sufferers have recurrent negative thoughts, many times a day. They imagine or worry that all sorts of really bad things will happen: 'I'll get AIDS', 'My house will burn down', or 'My children will die.' OCD sufferers are very distressed by these thoughts, and are often totally convinced that they will come true. But people start to recover from OCD when they realise that these thoughts will *not* actually come true. OCD sufferers have typically had these negative thoughts many thousands, if not millions of times – totally and utterly believing them – and yet they have never manifested in reality.

Another common idea is that negative thoughts are problematic because 'our thoughts control our actions'. If this were true, the human race would be in big trouble. After all, how often have you gotten so mad at somebody you care about that you thought about hurting in them some way – yelling at them, shaking them, leaving them or 'getting your own back'? (Be honest with yourself; we all have these thoughts at times.) Now just imagine if those thoughts *had* actually controlled you; if you *had* actually gone and done all those hurtful things. What would have happened to your closest relationships? Would you still have any friends left?

And have you ever thought about quitting, yet persisted? Have you ever thought of running away, but stayed and stuck it out? Clearly our thoughts don't control our actions. They certainly *influence* what we do, but they do not *control* what we do. And you'll soon discover how you can quickly reduce the influence of your negative thoughts, without even trying to get rid of them.

There is now a wealth of scientific studies, published in top peer-reviewed psychology journals, that show Acceptance and Commitment *Therapy* helps people to build rich, meaningful lives even in the face of serious conditions such as depression, schizophrenia, drug addiction and anxiety disorders. And in the worlds of business and sport, Acceptance and Commitment *Training* gets similar results: reducing stress, increasing fulfilment and enhancing performance. And yet, ACT makes no effort whatsoever to reduce, challenge, eliminate or change negative thoughts. Why not? Because ACT starts from the assumption that *negative thoughts are not inherently problematic.*

Now once again, just pause for ten seconds, and notice what your mind is saying.

***

So what did you hear? Something like, 'That can't be right', 'Is he serious?', 'I'm not buying it'? Or was it more like, 'Wow, that's interesting!' Whatever your mind is telling you, it's absolutely fine by me. Just let it chatter away, as if it's a radio playing in the background, and keep on reading.

To pick up where we left off: ACT assumes that *negative thoughts are not inherently problematic.* Negative thoughts only become problematic if we get all caught up in them, give them all our attention, treat them as the gospel truth, allow them to control us, or get into a fight with them. The technical term for responding to our thoughts in this way is 'fusion'.

Why 'fusion'? Well, think of two sheets of metal fused together. If you couldn't use the word 'fused' how would you describe them? Stuck, welded, bonded, melded, joined? These words all carry the same message: there is *no separation* between the sheets of metal. Similarly, when I talk about being fused with your thoughts, I mean there is no separation from them. In a state of fusion, we are completely 'entangled' by our thoughts: we are caught up in them, pushed around by them, lost in them, or fighting with them.

In other words, when we fuse with our thoughts, they have a huge impact on and influence over us. But when we 'defuse' from our thoughts – when we separate from them and realize that they are nothing more or less than words and pictures – then they have little or no effect on us (even if they happen to be true).

But don't take my word for it. In the next chapter, you will discover for yourself that no matter how 'negative' our thoughts are, they do not *have to* become problematic. When we know how to defuse from them, they lose their impact on and influence over us; they do not hold us back from being who we want to be, or doing what we want to do. You will discover that there is no need to fight with them, challenge them, suppress them, push them away, dwell on them or allow them to control you. All you need do is learn how to get yourself . . .

chapter 5

off the hook

Joe Simpson was freezing cold and in terrible agony; his right leg was broken, the knee completely shattered; and his climbing partner had left him for dead at the bottom of a huge crevasse.

He did not believe he was going to make it out alive. He had no food, water or fuel for a fire. He was lying on a bridge of ice, stranded on a deserted mountain in the Peruvian Andes. His climbing partner, convinced that Joe was dead, had gone back to base camp without him.

And yet, against all the odds, Joe managed to crawl out of the crevasse, dragging his mangled leg behind him, and make his way back to base camp. Although it was only six miles away, it took him three agonizing days to hop and crawl that distance.

You may know Joe's story from his awe-inspiring book, *Touching the Void*. One thing that struck me was that throughout his ordeal, Joe was bombarded by negative thoughts. He didn't have a head full of positive thoughts such as 'I will make it no matter what.' The odds were so overwhelmingly against him, he naturally believed he was going to die. But he did not let those thoughts stop him. He kept taking action, hauling his body, inch by inch, through the snow, even while his mind told him it was futile, he was as good as dead, and might as well give up.

Joe's story serves as a powerful reminder that negative thoughts need not hold us back. We don't have to wait until we're feeling all positive and optimistic. We can take action, even if our minds say we can't. Try this right now. Think to yourself, over and over, 'I can't lift my arm. I can't lift my arm' – and as you're thinking it, lift your arm up. Please do this now before reading on.

★★★

So there you go. You can lift your arm up even when your mind says that you can't. When I do this exercise in groups, I notice that many people hesitate for a second or two before they lift their arm up, and occasionally someone even takes a good ten or fifteen seconds. This is because we're used to taking our minds literally; to believing everything they tell us. Fortunately, we can learn to break this habit. We can learn how to do the things that really matter, even when our minds say it's not possible. We can learn the art of . . .

GETTING OFF THE HOOK

Have you ever seen a fish struggling to escape from a fishing line? No matter how hard it tries, its struggles are futile. Once it has swallowed that hook, it has no capacity to unhook itself.

In ACT, rather than using the technical term 'fusion', we often talk about 'getting hooked' by our thoughts. Our minds throw us thought after thought, inviting us to 'take the bait'. And if we bite, we 'get hooked'; we get all tangled up in our thoughts, and they exert a major influence over our actions. Fortunately, we can readily learn to 'unhook' ourselves (ie 'defuse' from our thoughts). And in this chapter, I'm going to take you through a range of simple techniques to show you how. But first, let's identify the types of thoughts that tend to hook us: all the various bits and pieces of the 'I can't do it' story that can so easily drag us away from doing what matters.

WHAT'S HOOKING YOU?

When you start thinking about making important changes – about being the person you want to be and doing the things you want to do – what sorts of things does your mind tend to say to you? Does it turn into a cheerleader and start singing some rousing motivational song such as:

'Go for it! You can do it! Knuckle on down and just get to it! It's so easy! Do it now! You've got the power! Ka-zam, ka-pow!'

I'm guessing that if you're anything like me, or the hundreds of clients I've worked with over the years, then about the only time your mind turns into a cheerleader is when your personal challenges are a long way off: 'Yes! I'll start it next year! Easy!' However, when you're staring that challenge directly in the face, it's a different story, isn't it?

Let me give you a peek into my world. As I'm writing the first draft of this chapter, early in the morning on a Saturday, I'm feeling a strong urge to quit. I am not in the mood for this. I am feeling spectacularly unmotivated, and I am sorely tempted right now to stop writing, and go and surf the internet, or answer some emails, or play with my son, or snack on a double-coated chocolate biscuit, or make a cup of tea; in other words, I want to do anything but write. My mind keeps saying things like, 'This is sooo boring', 'I'm not in the mood', 'It's too hard', 'I'll do it later', 'It's so warm and sunny outside, why not go for a lovely walk?', 'Your writing really sucks', 'This book's going to flop if you can't make it more interesting for your readers', 'Why don't you take a break and come back to it later?'

Now, what would happen if I were to get hooked by these thoughts? There are two likely outcomes: a) I'd stop writing; or b) I'd keep on plugging away, but instead of being focused and engaged in what I'm doing, I'd be all caught up in my thoughts, which would not only make writing difficult, but also impair the quality.

As it happens, both of these outcomes have happened to me many times. And sometimes they still do. You see, despite my best intentions, my mind still knows how to hook me. But the good news is, the more I practise, the better I get at unhooking myself, and the freer I am to do what truly matters to me. And that's why I am now writing my third book in under two years. (Believe me, if I had waited until my mind stopped being negative, then to this day I would not have written a word.)

So do you ever get hooked by thoughts a bit like mine? What effect does that have on you? Does it interfere with your performance, or hold you back from doing what you want to do? If so, good; that shows you you're a normal human being. That's what usually happens when people get hooked.

Below are some of the more common thoughts that hook us, and pull us away from achieving what we want. Which ones does your mind bait you with? (Add in any of your own that may be missing.)

'I've got no motivation', 'I've got no discipline', 'I've got no willpower', 'I'm too busy', 'I'm too tired', 'I don't have time', 'I don't have the energy', 'I'll start next week', 'I'll fail', 'It's a waste of time', 'I'll make a fool of myself', 'I don't have what it takes', 'I'm not ready', 'It's too hard', 'I need more practice', 'I need to read some more books about it', 'I need more equipment', 'Other people don't have to go through this', 'It shouldn't be this difficult', 'I'm too anxious' and 'Every time I've tried to change I've always failed so why should it be any different this time?'

I could easily fill up several more pages with thoughts and beliefs of this nature. Our minds are truly brilliant at coming up with reasons as to why we can't do what really matters to us. Thus, in ACT, we refer to all such thoughts as 'reason-giving'.

There are many different categories of 'reason-giving', but here are the four most common:

1. **Obstacles:** Our minds point out all those obstacles and difficulties that lie in our paths

2. **Self-judgements:** Our minds tell us all those ways in which we're not up to the task

3. **Comparisons:** Our minds compare us unfavourably to others who seem to do it better, have more talent, or have it easier

4. **Predictions:** Our minds predict failure, rejection or other unpleasant outcomes

In chapter 1 I mentioned Sarah, the unemployed dancer who said if she had more confidence she would attend more auditions and dance better in front of the judges. Sarah's mind was astonishingly creative; it managed to give her endless reasons not to go to auditions. It told her how awkward, embarrassed and anxious she would feel, how much practice she would have to do in order to get better, and how hard and boring and tedious that would be. It reminded her of all the hassle involved in getting to the locations by public transport, and then hanging around for ages, nerves jangling, waiting to be called in. It pointed out all the weaknesses in her dancing, and told her she was too lazy and didn't have the will-power or discipline to practise her routines. It compared her to other dancers she knew, and pointed out all the ways in which they were more athletic, graceful or talented. And it told her there was no point in trying because she was sure to fail anyway.

By the time Sarah came to see me, she was deeply frustrated. She had a veritable library of self-help books, and she'd followed their advice faithfully. She'd spent many, many hours challenging her negative thoughts, repeating positive affirmations, and visualizing herself stunning the judges with her dance moves. But it didn't stop her mind from churning out lots of reasons to avoid the auditions (or avoid practising her dance routines). We'll return to Sarah later in the chapter, but for now take a few moments to consider: which types of 'reason-giving' does your mind prefer? (My mind uses all of them!)

THE REASON-GIVING MACHINE

Our minds are like reason-giving machines; as soon as we think about making important changes, they crank out a whole list of reasons why we can't do it, shouldn't do it, or shouldn't *have to* do it. And there is no way to stop our minds from doing this. But don't take my word for it; check it out for yourself. Set yourself a goal right now – something you will do in the next few days that will take you out of your comfort zone into a genuinely challenging situation. (Obviously, pick something that is likely to improve your life; I don't mean anything dangerous like walking down a dark alleyway late at night.) If you have access to a pen and paper or a computer, then write your goal down. If not, just do it in your head. Please phrase your goal using this structure:

'My commitment is to take the following action: on . . . [specify the day, date and time here] I am going to . . . [specify here exactly what actions you will take with your arms, legs and mouth].'

Once you've done that, say your goal to yourself (aloud or silently) – and as you do so, notice what your mind starts telling you.

***

Did the reason-giving machine crank into action? Churning out all the reasons not to do it? I'd be surprised if it didn't – but that's easily fixed. To set the reason-giving machine in motion, all you need to do is up the stakes. Simply make a commitment right now that as soon as you finish this page, you will put the book down and publically announce your goal (either in person, via telephone or via email) to somebody whose opinion really matters to you.

Now listen in to your mind for twenty seconds, and notice all the reasons it comes up with.

***

If you did the above exercise, what tactics did you notice your mind using: obstacles, self-judgements, comparisons or predictions? If you didn't do it, please take a moment to reflect: your mind just gave you some reasons to skip the exercise – 'can't be bothered', 'do it later', 'can't think of anything right now', 'too hard', 'won't matter if I skip this bit' – and you got hooked! This is completely normal, by the way – many readers will have done the same thing as you. It just goes to show how good our minds are at reason-giving. (And now that you have that insight, please go back and do the exercise.)

BUT WHAT IF MY THOUGHTS ARE TRUE?

Sometimes when I first talk about reason-giving, my clients protest strongly: 'But these thoughts are *true*!' They are usually surprised when I reply, 'You know, in this approach, it's not about whether our thoughts are true or false. It's about whether they're *helpful*. If we allow these thoughts to guide our actions, will they help us to achieve the results we want? Will they help us to be the person we want to be? Will they help us to create the life we want to live?'

To make this clear, let's revisit the four most common categories of reason-giving:

1. Obstacles
Our minds point out all the obstacles and difficulties that lie in our paths.

We all have obstacles, barriers and difficulties that get in the way of us doing the things we want to do. And our minds are very effective problem-solving machines. So if your mind is realistically appraising those obstacles and constructively figuring out how to overcome them, then such thoughts are likely to be helpful. For example, suppose the barrier or difficulty is lack of time, and your mind says, 'Yes, I am very busy. So to make time to practise my presentation skills, I'll cut back on the amount of TV I watch.' Thoughts like this are likely to be helpful. But if your mind just keeps going over and over all the potential obstacles, complaining about them, shoving them in your face, and telling you how hard it all is, without looking for constructive, practical solutions, then those thoughts are likely to be unhelpful.

2. Self-judgements
Our minds point out all those ways in which we're not up to the task.

Our minds are good at spotting what can be improved upon. So if our minds are respectfully appraising our skills, and constructively advising us as to how we can improve them, that's generally useful. For example, if your mind says, 'I'm not very good at telling jokes, and I'd like to improve, so I'm going to buy a joke book and practise telling jokes to my trusted friends,' that's probably helpful. But if your mind just criticizes and judges you – 'I'm hopeless at socializing. I can't tell jokes for the life of me. I always get flustered and forget the punchline' – that's unhelpful.

3. Comparisons
Our minds compare us unfavourably to others who seem to do it better, have more talent, or have it easier.

The mind is very good at making comparisons. Sometimes it tells us the ways in which we are 'better' than others, and sometimes it tells us the ways in which we are 'worse'. If our minds compare us to others in a respectful and constructive way that allows us to learn, grow and develop, that's generally helpful. Suppose your mind says, 'Tiger Woods can play golf much better than I can. What sorts of things does he do to improve his game? How much practice does he do? How can I emulate some of those strategies?' Allowing those thoughts to guide us will probably be helpful. But if your mind just blathers on about how others are so much better than you are, or how much easier they've got it, then that's not likely to be of much use.

4. Predictions
Our minds predict failure, rejection or other unpleasant outcomes.

As you know, our minds evolved to warn us of danger; to anticipate anything that could harm us. So when your mind starts predicting failure or disaster, it's only doing its job. Now suppose it does this in a constructive manner: realistically appraising the risks, planning how to respond in the worst-case scenario, and reminding us how we can learn from the experience. For example: 'Yes, it's true, if I write this book there's no guarantee that it will get published. The fact is, many books don't. And even if it does get published, most books make very little money. The odds of it being a bestseller are millions to one. But at least if I write it, I stand a chance. If I don't write it, I stand no chance at all. And in the worst-case scenario, even if it never gets published, I have the satisfaction of knowing I gave it my best shot. Plus, I got to improve my creative writing skills.' Thoughts like this are likely to be helpful. If we let them guide us, they'll take us in the direction we want to go. But if your mind is just broadcasting doom and gloom – 'There's no point starting. It'll never get published. It's a waste of time.' – then letting those thoughts guide you is probably unhelpful.

Notice, in each example above, the helpful thoughts did not involve 'reason-giving' – coming up with all the reasons why we 'can't do it'. Instead they provided constructive advice on what we *can* do.

Now once again, pause for a few seconds, and notice what your mind has to say about 'reason-giving'.

***

Is your mind objecting? Is it saying, 'But what if you really can't do it? What if you want to ride a bike but you have no legs?' Obviously, if there is a genuinely insurmountable obstacle, you will need to change your goal to a more realistic one. But fortunately, this is rarely the case. We can overcome most of our obstacles – even if our minds insist that we can't. To quote Nelson Mandela: 'It always seems impossible until it's done.'

A VERY IMPORTANT WORD

At this point, I'd like to introduce one of the most important words in this book: 'workability'. Please etch this word deep into your brain, as it underpins everything we do from this point onwards.

The term 'workability' arises from this simple question: 'Is what you are doing working to help you create a richer, fuller, more meaningful life?' If the answer is 'yes', then what you are doing is 'workable'. If the answer is 'no', then what you are doing is 'unworkable'.

The concept of workability can help us to unhook from our thoughts. If your aim is to empower yourself so you can take effective action and be who you really want to be, but your mind is generating all sorts of reasons as to why that just can't happen, then you can ask yourself this question: 'If I allow this thought to guide my actions, will it help me create the life I want?' If the answer is 'no', then you can recognize that the thought is 'unhelpful' and acting on it would be 'unworkable'. It only takes a few seconds to do this: to pause, check in, notice what your mind is saying, and ask yourself the question above. Recognizing a thought or belief as unhelpful often helps to reduce its influence over us; it makes us less likely to act on it. However, note that with this approach, we're not getting into debates about whether the thought is true or false; the question we're interested in is simply this: 'If I let this thought dictate my actions, will it help me to lead the life I want?'

A MULTITUDE OF METHODS

I'm now going to take you through a whole stack of different defusion techniques (the first three all come from Steven Hayes' first ACT textbook, *Acceptance and Commitment Therapy: An experiential approach to behaviour change*) so you can discover which ones best help you to unhook. Some of them may seem a bit weird or wacky, but please give them a go and see what happens. In each case, I'll ask you first to fuse with the thought (i.e. buy into it, give it all your attention, believe it as much as you can), so you can get yourself well and truly hooked. Then I'll help you to unhook again.

Before we embark, a word of caution: there's no technique in the whole of psychology that always achieves the desired result. While most people find these techniques help them to detach, separate, or get some distance from their thoughts, occasionally the opposite may occur: you may find that the thought starts reeling you in! So adopt an attitude of curiosity towards these exercises; let go of your expectations and just see what happens. Notice whether the technique helps you to separate from the thought (defusion) or whether it seems to draw you in even closer (fusion).

(Note: fusion isn't likely to happen with these exercises; I'm just warning you about it on the off-chance that it does. If it does, please regard it as a learning opportunity: a chance for you to notice what it's like to get hooked. Then move on to the next exercise.)

For each exercise, read the instructions through first, then give it a go. And if a particular technique does not work for you, or you simply can't do it, then move on to the next.

Exercise 1: I'm having the thought that . . .
Bring to mind a thought that readily hooks you, and pulls you away from the life you want to live. Ideally, for this exercise pick a negative self-judgement that plays a key role in the 'I can't do it' story – eg 'I'm not smart enough', or 'I don't have what it takes' or 'I'm a loser.'

- Silently say this thought to yourself, believing it as much as you can, and notice the effect it has on you.
- Now replay that thought in your head, with this short phrase inserted immediately before it: 'I'm having the thought that . . .' For example, 'I'm having the thought that I'm a loser.'

- Now replay that thought once more, but this time the phrase to insert is: 'I notice I'm having the thought that . . .' For example, 'I notice I'm having the thought that I'm a loser.'

So what happened? Most people get a sense of distance or separation from the thought. If this didn't happen for you, please try again with another self-judgement. (And if you didn't do the exercise at all, please note the reasons your mind gave you to skip it, then go back and do it anyway.)

Exercise 2: Singing thoughts
Use the same negative self-judgement as above, or if it has lost its impact, pick a different one.
- Silently say this thought to yourself, believing it as much as you can, and notice what effect it has on you.
- Now replay this thought, word for word the same, singing it to the tune of 'Happy Birthday'. (You can either sing it silently or aloud.)
- Now replay that thought once more, but this time, sing it to the tune of your choice.

What happened this time? Most people find the sense of distance or separation from the thought is greater than with the first exercise. Some people even find themselves smiling or chuckling, however that's not the point of the exercise. The point is, when we hear our thoughts sung to music, it helps us to see their true nature: just like the lyrics in a song, our thoughts are nothing more nor less than *words*. (Of course, thoughts can also occur in the form of pictures or images, but for now we're just dealing with words.)

Exercise 3: Silly voices

Use the same negative self-judgement as above, or if it has lost its impact, pick a different one.

- Silently say this thought to yourself, believing it as much as you can.
- Now replay it, word for word the same, hearing it in the voice of a cartoon character, movie star or sports commentator.
- Now replay it again in yet another distinctive voice, for example that of a posh English actor or a sitcom character.

This technique is similar to singing our thoughts. When we hear our thoughts said in different voices, again it helps us to separate from them – and recognise that they are nothing more nor less than words.

Exercise 4: Computer screen

Use the same negative self-judgement as above, or if it has lost its impact, pick a different one.

- Silently say this thought to yourself, believing it as much as you can.
- Now close your eyes, imagine a computer, and see this thought as words on the screen, written in simple black text.
- Now play around with the font and the colour of the text. Don't change the words themselves; just see them in three or four different colours, and three or four different fonts.
- Now put the words back into simple black text, and this time, play around with the formatting. First, space the words out – large gaps between them.

- Now run all the words together – no gaps between them.
- Now run the words vertically down the screen, underneath each other.
- Finally, put the words back into simple black text, and this time add in a karaoke ball, bouncing from word to word, back and forth. And if you like, just for good measure, also sing the thought to the tune of your choice.

This exercise tends to be more effective for more 'visual' people. Again, hopefully it helped you to separate or distance from your thought: to see that it is constructed out of words.

Now, once again tune in to your mind, and for ten seconds, notice what it's telling you.

***

So how's your mind reacting? Maybe it's excited: 'Wow! That was amazing!' Or maybe it's all worked up: 'How can he say that thoughts are "just words"? They're true!', 'This guy is patronizing me', 'He doesn't get how it is for me; he doesn't understand the way these thoughts kick me around.' Or maybe it's a bit disappointed: 'These techniques are just silly tricks, they're not going to help me.'

Whatever your mind is doing, please allow it to have its reaction. And if that reaction is particularly strong and unhelpful, then I invite you to try something. It's a little technique, developed by Steve Hayes, called 'thanking your mind'. Whatever your mind says – no matter how provocative, nasty or scary it may be – you silently reply, with a sense of humour, 'Thanks mind.' You can of course vary this as desired, for example, 'Thanks for sharing' or 'Thanks mind, good story.' Personally, it's one of my favourite defusion exercises, so play around with it and see what you think. Remember, we're not trying to stop our minds from having these reactions; this technique is simply to help us detach from those thoughts.

THE POWER OF WORDS

You've probably heard the quotation, 'The pen is mightier than the sword.' This saying succinctly reminds us that words can have an enormous influence over our behaviour. For example, books, scriptures and manifestos can, in certain situations, shape entire nations far more powerfully than violence, bloodshed and warfare.

Likewise, in a state of fusion, those words inside our heads can have a huge impact upon us. They can dredge up panic or despair; they can feel like a kick in the guts or a plank on our chest; they can drag us down into the depths and sap all our strength.

However, in a state of defusion, our thoughts are nothing more nor less than words. Hopefully you got to experience that, at least to some degree, in the previous exercises. If you didn't, no matter; we'll be doing some more defusion very soon.

In ACT, we do not belittle your challenges or patronize you; we don't try to deny the powerful impact that thoughts can have on our actions. We simply aim to empower you; to increase the choices available to you in your life. Once we can defuse from our thoughts – i.e. separate from them and see them for what they are – we have many more options in life. No longer are we at the mercy of our minds, pushed around by ingrained patterns of unhelpful automatic thinking. Instead we can choose to pursue what truly matters to us – even when our minds make it hard with all that reason-giving.

IF YOUR HANDS WERE YOUR THOUGHTS

Many people misunderstand the point of defusion. They either think it's a way to get rid of negative thoughts, or a way to control your feelings. But it's neither. Here's an exercise to clarify what it's for. To do this, you'll need to position the book in such a way that you can read the instructions while keeping both your hands free to do the exercise. For example, you might spread it flat on a desktop, and use a paperweight to keep the pages open. Alternatively, you could memorize the instructions, or have someone else read them out to you.

- In this exercise, pretend that your hands are your thoughts.
- Place them in front of you, palms upwards, side-by-side – as if they were the open pages of a book.
- Ever so slowly, raise them up towards your face.
- Gradually bring them closer, until they are covering your eyes.
- Keeping your hands over your eyes, look at the world around you. How much are you missing out on? Imagine going around all day like this. How hard would it be to act effectively and do the things that make your life work?
- Now, ever so slowly, lower your hands.
- As the gap between your hands and face increases, notice what happens. How much better is your view of the world around you? How much more information can you take in? How much more effectively can you act?
- Now let your hands rest. Notice they have not disappeared. They are still with you. If there's some way you can use them to improve your life, you are free to use them. If there's nothing they're useful for right now,

you can give them some space to rest and just let
them be.

So here you see the two main purposes of defusion. Firstly, it enables us to 'be present': to connect with the world around us, and engage in whatever we are doing. Secondly, it enables us to take effective action. Obviously if our thoughts are helpful, we will make use of them. But if they're not, we'll just give them plenty of space and let them be.

To develop genuine confidence, we need to be fully present and engaged in whatever we are doing – whether it's playing golf, giving a speech, making conversation or making love. And we also need to be capable of effective action. Defusion enables both of these things.

So why do some people get totally the wrong idea? Why do they think defusion is a clever way to get rid of negative thoughts? Because very often, when we defuse from a thought, it disappears. And often, over time, it shows up with lesser frequency. However, this is just a bonus; it's a by-product of defusion, not the main purpose.

Other people mistake defusion as a way to control unpleasant feelings. Why? Because often when we defuse from negative thoughts, we feel better, calmer or happier. But again, this is just a lucky bonus, not the main aim; and it certainly won't always happen. The purpose of defusion is this: to be present and take effective action.

So here's my guarantee: if you start using defusion techniques to try to get rid of negative thoughts or to control how you feel, you'll soon be disappointed or frustrated. Why? Well, firstly, it won't work. Sure, it may work as a quick-fix technique in an unchallenging situation, but once you get into the real-life challenging situation, it will not have the desired effect. Secondly, if you're trying to control how you feel, then you've once again gotten stuck inside 'the confidence gap'. Once again, you're playing by the wrong rules: *I have to feel confident before I do what matters;* or *I have to get rid of negative thoughts, and reduce my fear or anxiety, before I can behave like the person I want to be.*

So one more time, for good measure: the purpose of defusion is to help us be present and take effective action. This gives us the third rule for the confidence game:

Rule 3: 'Negative' thoughts are normal. Don't fight them; defuse them.

THE POWER OF PRACTICE

I've said it before and I'll say it again: improving our lives requires committed action. That often means learning new skills or working on old ones. And obviously, if we want to become skilful at *anything*, we need to practise. This goes for psychological skills as well as physical ones. We can't develop good defusion skills without practice. And we all need these skills, because the reason-giving machine is here to stay. It's not going to suddenly transform into your own personal cheerleader or motivational guru. It's going to keep on telling you multiple versions of the 'I can't do it' story. So are you willing to practise the techniques in this chapter?

What I'm asking you to do is very simple. The moment you notice you've been hooked by an unworkable thought, acknowledge it. Silently say to yourself, 'Just got hooked!' Then replay the thought using any technique you like: I'm Having the Thought That, Singing Thoughts, Silly Voices or The Computer Screen. (And keep in mind, these techniques are like training wheels on a bicycle. You won't have to go for the rest of your life singing your thoughts to 'Happy Birthday' or hearing them in the voice of Homer Simpson. This is just a convenient place to start.)

I invite you to do this as an experiment; to let go of any expectations you may have, and bring an attitude of genuine curiosity to your experience. Notice what happens, or doesn't happen. Don't expect any miraculous overnight changes. And if you do notice high expectations popping up, then gently unhook yourself; for example, you might say, 'I'm having the thought that this should magically solve all my problems.'

At times you may be hooked for hours before you realize it – worrying, ruminating, over-analysing or 'stressing out'. No problem. The moment you realise you're hooked, gently acknowledge it: 'Hooked again!' Then pick the thought that's hooking you the most, and replay it with the technique of your choice.

So are you willing to give it a go? Just pause for ten seconds, and again notice what your mind is saying.

***

What's it doing this time? Is it all revved up and eager to practise? Or is it cranking out reasons not to do it: 'It's too silly', 'It won't work', 'I'll do it later', 'I can't be bothered', 'It doesn't really matter' and so on. If the latter, no surprises there! Let your mind try its best to dissuade you – then do it anyway. And if you should at some point find yourself hooked by all that reason-giving, then you know the drill: acknowledge 'Just got hooked!', then do a replay.

I recommend you use these techniques at least five times a day, to begin with; the more the better. And if you don't use them, notice how your mind talked you out of it: did it come up with some really good new reasons, or did it pull out the same old ones it's been using for years?

The good thing is, you'll have plenty of material to practise with, because your mind is . . .

chapter 6

never short of words

Poisonous black smoke drifts over the city. The people see it and run towards the river . . . thousands of them, jumping into it like rats. And those that run too slowly start dropping like flies.

At least, that's how they described it on the radio. On 30 October 1938, CBS Radio broadcast a programme called *The War of the Worlds*, a dramatization of H.G. Wells' famous novel about Martians invading Earth. The one-hour episode was written, directed and narrated by the up-and-coming actor Orson Welles. The first two-thirds of the show consisted of fake news bulletins: 'reporters' describing the Martian attacks, 'live from the scene'. Many listeners missed the start of the show, and so failed to realize that it was only a radio play. They heard the 'breaking news' and thought the Martians really were attacking. Mass panic ensued.

The next day, the *New York Times* reported:

In Newark, in a single block at Heddon Terrace and Hawthorne

> *Avenue, more than twenty families rushed out of their houses with wet handkerchiefs and towels over their faces to flee from what they believed was to be a gas raid. Some began moving household furniture. Throughout New York families left their homes, some to flee to nearby parks. Thousands of persons called the police, newspapers and radio stations here and in other cities of the United States and Canada, seeking advice on protective measures against the raids.*

To listeners who knew the show was just a play, the words coming out of the radio were not a problem. But for listeners who took the words literally, the experience was terrifying. This provides a good analogy for the point I made in the previous chapter: that the words inside our head are not a problem; the problem lies in the way we respond to them. If we fuse with those words, they can easily cause us difficulties. But if we defuse, they don't. (If you've been practising the techniques from the previous chapter, you'll know what I'm talking about.)

In some ways, the mind is like a radio; have you noticed how it's always got something to say? It's always got an opinion, an idea, a prediction, a judgement, a criticism, a comparison or a complaint. It's like listening to talkback radio all day long. Sure, from time to time it quietens down – but it soon starts up again, doesn't it? Blah, blah, blah, blah, blah. It doesn't even stop broadcasting when we're asleep. However, this similarity to a radio gives us a simple method for unhooking ourselves.

RADIO TRIPLE F

It's time to revisit your Life Change List from chapter 1 (the list of what you'll do differently as you develop confidence). Now pick one of the things on that list, and for a few seconds, imagine starting to do it *today*. No matter how tiny the step you take – writing the opening line of that novel, downloading the enrolment form for that course, rehearsing what you'll say when you ask that special person out on a date – imagine yourself taking that first step today. Do this now for about thirty seconds.

★★★

Now stop and notice: what is your mind doing? Is it 'reason-giving'? Telling you the 'I can't do it' story? If your mind is being very positive, enjoy it; most readers, though, will find that their minds are saying something unhelpful.

Now what if your mind really were a radio station? For many people, it would sound a little bit like this: 'Welcome to Radio Triple F: Fear, Flaws and Failure. Regular bulletins on everything you need to fear! Keeping you updated on all your flaws! Around-the-clock reminders about failure! We're here for you all day, every day.'

If this sounds a bit like your mind, good! That's a sign that you have a normal human mind. Of course, it doesn't *always* broadcast doom and gloom. At times it can be very helpful, and later in the book we'll look at how to use it to our advantage – not with 'positive' thinking but with 'effective' thinking. But for now, let's face reality: our minds evolved to think negatively! And the bigger and more immediate the challenges we face, the more likely we are to hear 'Radio Triple F'.

So how can we unhook ourselves?

The first step is simply to notice we've been hooked. The second step is to name what's going on. A sense of humour can really help here. For example, we could say: 'Aha! Here's Radio Triple F broadcasting again.' Or just 'Radio Triple F'. Or simply 'Oops. Hooked again.'

Often these two steps give us enough defusion from our thoughts for us to re-engage in the world and do what matters. However, we can defuse even further if desired. A third step is to imagine that your mind is a radio, and your thoughts are like a voice coming out through the speakers. You could even hear the thoughts in the voice of your favourite newsreader or sports commentator. (And recognise that you've heard this broadcast many times!)

Why not try this out right now? Remember that Life Change List from chapter 1: ways you want to act differently, things you want to do differently, goals you want to achieve, and so on. Read through the list now, or go back to that chapter and remind yourself of your answers. Then pick something on the list that you can make a start on immediately. Think of some small, simple actions you can take today that would get you moving in the direction you want to go.

Once you've done that, just pause . . . and for twenty seconds, notice what your mind is doing.

***

So what's your mind telling you? If it's being helpful, fantastic; go and get started! But if your mind is being unhelpful, try this technique out right now: a) notice what your mind is saying; b) name it: 'Here's Radio Triple F'; c) hear your thoughts as if they were coming from a radio.

***

So what happened? If you didn't find it much use, not to worry. There are hundreds of other defusion techniques. You can even invent your own, as we'll see.

THREE STEPS TO DEFUSION

All defusion techniques involve one or more of the following steps. When a thought hooks us, we can:

1.   Notice it
2.   Name it
3.   Neutralize it

Let's quickly look at each step.

1. Notice it

Noticing our thoughts is always the first step in defusion, and often it's enough to do the job by itself. If you pause for a second and notice what your mind is doing, that opens a little space between you and your thoughts; often enough for them to lose some of their influence over you.

2. Name it

When we name the type of thoughts we're having, that often helps us to defuse from them. There are many ways to do this. You tried a couple of techniques in the previous chapter: 'Aha! Here's reason-giving!' or 'Here's the "I can't do it" story', or 'I'm having the thought that . . .' You can silently say anything to yourself that names this particular pattern of thinking. For example, if you catch yourself worrying, you may say 'Worrying again'. If you catch yourself imagining the worst, you may say 'Imagining the worst'. If you catch yourself getting caught up in negative self-judgements, you may say 'Judging again'.

It's more effective if you can do this with a sense of humour; as if you are smiling in recognition, giving yourself a knowing wink: 'Aha. Just got hooked again!'

You can also use metaphors to name your thinking. For example, if your mind is trying to boss you around like a fascist dictator, you might say to yourself, 'There goes the fascist dictator.' Or if your mind is being very pessimistic, you might say 'Ah, yes. Mr Doom-and-Gloom is on the podium.'

3. Neutralize it

This is an optional step that gives room for a huge amount of creativity. I use the word 'neutralize' to mean take your thoughts and put them into a new context, where you can see them clearly for what they are: nothing more than pictures and words; nothing you need to fight with, cling to or run from.

In the previous chapter you did this in several different ways: silently singing your thoughts, hearing them in silly voices, putting them on to a computer screen. And in this chapter you've imagined them as a broadcast on the radio. However, there are dozens, if not hundreds, of ways to do this. Here are a few ideas to stimulate your creative juices. I encourage you to play around with them, see how they work for you, and see if you can come up with some of your own.

You could visualize the thought as a caption on a birthday card, or a slogan on a T-shirt, or graffiti on a wall. You could say the thought aloud in a squeaky voice or a foreign accent, or sing it to the tune of your choice. You might write it down, draw it or paint it; or perhaps imagine yourself painting it on a canvas. You might visualise your thoughts as the credits of a movie, scrolling up the screen (or maybe even floating through space, as in the *Star Wars* movies). You can place your thoughts on clouds, and let them drift across the sky; or put them on to suitcases on a conveyor belt. You could imagine an actor reading your thoughts from a script. Or you could imagine them as text messages, emails or pop-ups on the internet.

And if you came up with a metaphor in step 2, such as the fascist dictator, or Mr Doom-and-Gloom in step 3, you could take it further. You might actually imagine a fascist dictator saying your thoughts out loud, giving a speech to a crowd of fanatic followers. Or you might imagine Mr Doom-and-Gloom as a character in a comic book, and see your thoughts popping up inside his speech bubbles. Basically, you can do anything that helps you step back and see that thoughts are nothing more or less than 'mental events': constructions of words and pictures; transient and ever-changing.

THE 'P' WORD

I encourage you to play with defusion throughout the day; to get better and better at unhooking yourself. Remember, if we want to become good at anything, there's no getting away from the need to practise. So, as well as practising these ultra-quick defusion exercises, I invite you to try a longer one, also by Steven Hayes, called 'leaves on a stream'. Ideally you'd practise this for five to ten minutes, once or twice a day; the more the better. Many people find it works well to slot five, ten or fifteen minutes into a lunch break, or to do it first thing in the morning, as soon as they're out of bed.

Please read through the instructions at least *twice*, then give it a go. (And if you'd like a recording of this exercise to help guide you through it, you'll find it on track two of my CD, *Mindfulness Skills: Volume 1,* available as a CD or MP3 from www.thehappinesstrap. co.uk.)

LEAVES ON A STREAM

Note: if you have difficulty visualizing (i.e. creating images and pictures inside your head) then you will need to modify this exercise. You'll find out how as you read on.

1. Find a comfortable position, sitting or lying, and either close your eyes or fix them on a spot.
2. Imagine a gently flowing stream.
3. Imagine there are leaves floating on the surface of the water.
4. For the next five minutes, take every thought that

pops into your head – whether it's a picture or a word – place it on top of a leaf, and let it float on by.

5.   If you find visualization hard, or you can't get the stream to look the way you want it to, then instead imagine an expanse of black space. And imagine there's a gently blowing breeze. Take each thought that pops into your head, release it into the breeze, and let it float off into the blackness. Alternatively, you could imagine a moving black strip, like a conveyor belt, and place your thoughts on that.

6.   Do this for each and every thought, whether it is happy or sad, positive or negative, optimistic or pessimistic. You may find yourself trying to 'hold on' to the happy, positive, optimistic thoughts. If so, remember the purpose of the exercise is to improve your ability at unhooking yourself, at 'letting go' of your thoughts, so if you want to get good at this, you need to practise on *every* thought that arises, both pleasant and unpleasant, helpful and unhelpful. (Not for the rest of your life; just while doing this exercise.)

7.   You are not aiming to get rid of the thoughts. You are aiming to 'step back' and watch their natural flow. (So, if you start speeding up the stream, trying to wash them all away, you are defeating the purpose.)

8.   If your thoughts stop, watch the stream (or the blackness). It won't be long before they start again.

9.   If your mind says, 'This is silly' or 'It's too hard' or 'I can't do it', put those thoughts on to leaves too.

10.   Most people get hooked early on by thoughts like 'I'm not doing it properly', or 'It's flowing too fast', or 'I can't get the stream to look how I want.' When you notice you've been hooked by such a thought,

simply restart the exercise, and put that thought on to a leaf.

11. If a leaf or a thought 'gets stuck' and doesn't move on, let it stay. Don't fight with it. Sometimes thoughts hang around for a while before they eventually move on.

12. If an uncomfortable feeling shows up, like boredom, frustration, impatience or anxiety, just acknowledge it. Silently say to yourself 'Noticing boredom' or 'Noticing frustration'. And then place those words on to a leaf.

13. From time to time you'll get hooked and pulled out of the exercise: you'll get stuck planning your holidays, or running through your to-do list, or rehashing that quarrel you recently had with your partner, or thinking about that movie you saw last night, or remembering that stream you used to play in as a child. This is only natural; our minds are experts at hooking us. The moment you realise you've been hooked, silently acknowledge it: 'Hooked again'. Then start up the exercise again from the beginning.

Please read the above instructions as many times as you need to until you know what to do, then give it a go. Five minutes is ideal for a first run-through, but you can do more or less as you desire.

★★★

So how did you find that? (Did you actually do it, or did the 'reason-giving' machine get the better of you?) Did you get repeatedly hooked and pulled out of the exercise? If so, that's absolutely normal, and only to be expected. Our minds are very creative; they have many different ways of interfering – and not just with this exercise, with all of them! However, each time you realize you've been hooked, and proceed to unhook yourself again, you are developing a valuable skill.

People have a wide range of reactions to this exercise. Some folks love it; others hate it; most lie somewhere in between. I did not like it very much at first, but I found that after a couple of weeks of daily practice, I came to enjoy it. Many of my clients have found the same. So I encourage you to persist, at least for a week or two. And how will this practice help you develop confidence? Let's think it through.

JUST IMAGINE . . .

You've done it. You've taken the plunge. You've stepped out of your comfort zone and put yourself into that challenging situation. You're about to give that talk, or ask that person for a date, or write the first sentence of that book. You're mingling at the party, waiting for the whistle to start the game, or waiting to go through that door for your big interview.

Your fight-or-flight-response has kicked in, and your mind is now going into a tailspin. Maybe it's predicting disaster. Maybe it's telling you that you can't handle it. Maybe it's simply piling on the pressure, warning you of what's at stake, and what could go wrong. And yet . . . it's not a problem. Those thoughts just float on by, like leaves on a stream. You don't have to challenge them, or squash them. You just let them come and go, as if they were merely cars, driving past outside your house.

And because you're not investing any effort in fighting them, disputing them, or suppressing them, you can now put your energy into taking effective action. And because you're not entangled in your thoughts, you can engage fully in whatever it is that you're doing.

Of course, we wouldn't practise 'leaves on a stream' while we're in the middle of a challenging situation, or we wouldn't be able to act effectively. 'Leaves on a stream' is merely a training exercise to help develop the skill of defusion. Once this skill is developed, we can go into challenging situations and defuse from our thoughts spontaneously, without needing to rely on such techniques.

Remember Sarah, the dancer we spoke about in chapter 5? In the past, whenever she attended an audition, she'd get so entangled in thoughts of failure, she'd be unable to focus on what she was doing. As a result, she wouldn't dance very well, and she'd fail the audition: a self-fulfilling prophecy. However, once she started practising 'leaves on a stream' every day for twenty minutes, she soon noticed a huge difference. At auditions, her mind would still generate plenty of thoughts about failure, but she was able to let them come and go without getting wrapped up in them. She could focus on her routine, and danced much better. Did this help her self-confidence? You bet it did!

Now pause for twenty seconds, and notice what your mind is telling you.

***

Is the reason-giving machine cranking up? Is Radio Triple F doing a broadcast? Is your mind telling you some version of the 'I can't do it' story? If so, no surprises there. So thank your mind for those thoughts and carry on reading.

On the other hand, if your mind is being positive and encouraging, enjoy it. Remember, the mind is a double-edged sword. At times, it *will* generate thoughts that are helpful; and at other times it will do the very opposite. And sometimes it will even do both simultaneously. So enjoy it when your mind is being helpful – but don't come to rely on it, because it can change like the wind. And especially be alert for . . .

chapter 7

the self-esteem trap

In the great Wall Street Crash of 1929, bankrupt business-men leapt from the rooftops of their buildings. And in 2009 Michael knew exactly how they felt.

One year earlier, Michael had been the director of a hugely prof-itable company. But now, everything had changed. The global financial crisis had crippled his business, and he was now forced to sell it at a major loss.

Michael was in a truly wretched state. Miserable, hopeless and defeated – a far cry from how he'd felt twelve months earlier. When he had been doing well, at the top of his game, he thought of himself as a 'winner'. And not surprisingly, that made him feel good. But now the tide had turned. Now his mind kept telling him he was a 'loser'. And that, surprise, surprise, did *not* feel so good. Michael was painfully caught in the 'self-esteem trap'.

FALLING INTO THE TRAP
Our society often encourages us to think in terms of 'winners' and

'losers', 'successes' and 'failures', 'champions' and 'underachievers'. We frequently encounter all sorts of books, articles and experts that tell us: 'Think like a winner!', 'Be a success', 'Winners do this!' and 'Losers do that!'

If we get hooked by the story that we're a 'winner', a 'champion' or a 'success', there may well be some short-term benefits. For example, we may get to feel good about ourselves for a while. (Especially if we compare ourselves to some 'loser', 'failure' or 'quitter'.) But how long does that feeling last? How long before our minds find someone else who is achieving more or being 'more successful' than us?

And when our minds inevitably locate that other person and start comparing, what happens next? That's right: now our minds call us the 'loser' or 'failure'.

You may have heard of the concept of 'fragile self-esteem'. It's something very common in 'successful' professionals and athletes. As long as they achieve all their goals, they can hold on tightly to the 'I'm a winner' story, and they get to feel good about themselves. But the moment their performance drops – and sooner or later, it will – the story instantly changes to 'I'm a loser'. And if they're in the habit of holding on tight to self-judgements, then they get reeled in to the black hole of 'I'm a loser'.

So the 'winners/losers' mindset is inherently problematic. It creates a desperate need to achieve, fuelled by the fear of becoming a 'loser' or a 'failure'. This in turn leads to chronic stress, performance anxiety or burnout.

And consider this too: when someone holds on tightly to 'I'm a winner', in the long term, what effect does that have on their relationships? Have you ever tried to build a good-quality relationship, based on openness, respect and equality, with someone hooked on their own positive self-judgements; someone completely fused with 'I am a success', 'I am a champion' or 'I am a winner'?

We read all the time about rock stars, movie stars, supermodels and other famous people who take their own press too seriously and start to believe they really are better than everyone else, and we see how much tension and stress they create with their narcissistic, egocentric behaviour. Contrast these folks with Nelson Mandela, who said in one interview: 'That was one of the things that worried me – to be raised to the position of a semi-god – because then you are no longer a human being. I wanted to be known as Mandela, a man with weaknesses – some of which are fundamental.'

THE SELF-ESTEEM MYTH

The self-esteem industry is worth a small fortune, and it has done an excellent job of selling us on the importance of its products. Once a term used only by psychologists, 'self-esteem' is now a household word, with parents, teachers, therapists and coaches preaching its many benefits. But does high self-esteem live up to its own reputation? Does it really make us happier, healthier and more successful? Or have we all been hoodwinked by a seductive sales pitch?

First, let's define what 'high self-esteem' actually means, because there is more than one interpretation. By far the most common meaning of 'high self-esteem' is evaluating oneself positively; in other words, making *and believing* positive self-judgements and self-appraisals. (This is often described as prizing, appreciating or approving of oneself.) Now keeping to this popular meaning of the term, please do the following quiz. Answer each statement true or false:

- Boosting your self-esteem will improve your performance.
- People with high self-esteem are more likeable, have better relationships, and make a better impression on others.
- People with high self-esteem make better leaders.

Before I give you the answers, let's go back in time to 2003. In that year, the American Psychological Association commissioned a 'Self-esteem Task Force' to investigate if the claims above (and many other similar ones) were true. So a team of four psychologists from top universities – Roy Baumeister, Jennifer Campbell, Joachim Krueger and Kathleen Vohs – systematically ploughed through decades of published research on self-esteem. They looked long and hard for firm scientific evidence to either confirm or refute these popular beliefs. Then they published their results in an influential journal called *Psychological Science in the Public Interest*. And what did they find? All three of the above statements are false!

They also found that:

- High self-esteem correlates with egotism, narcissism and arrogance.
- High self-esteem correlates with prejudice and discrimination.
- High self-esteem correlates with self-deception and defensiveness when faced with honest feedback.

And as if this news weren't bad enough by itself, cast your mind back to the research I cited in chapter 3: when people with *low* self-esteem try to boost it through positive self-affirmations, they generally end up feeling even worse!

So if trying to raise self-esteem is not worth the effort, then what's the alternative?

SELF-ACCEPTANCE

Self-acceptance, self-awareness and self-motivation are all far more important than self-esteem. (For now, we're going to focus on self-acceptance; we'll cover the others in later chapters.)

Why is self-acceptance so important? Because when we step out of our comfort zones, things won't always turn out the way we desire. At times we will make mistakes and screw things up. At other times things will go wrong when we least expect it. And although sometimes we will achieve our goals quite easily, sometimes we are bound to fail dismally. This is a fact of life, no matter how talented or dedicated we may be. Michael Jordan, commonly acclaimed as the greatest basketball player of all time, provides a good example:

> *I've missed more than 9,000 shots in my career. I've lost almost 300 games. Twenty-six times I've been trusted to take the game winning shot . . . and missed. I've failed over and over and over again in my life. That is why I succeed.*

We can easily agree with this intellectually. 'Yes,' we can say, 'that makes good sense. Making mistakes is an essential part of the learning process.' However, when it actually happens, when we *really do* screw up, our minds are generally not so agreeable. At these times, the mind's 'default setting' is to beat us up; to pull out a big stick and give us a whacking.

Now, here's the million-dollar question: if beating yourself up were a good way to change your behaviour, wouldn't you be perfect by now? Just think back over all the floggings, hidings and beatings your mind has doled out over your lifetime. Did they really help you? Or did they just make you feel bad? And even if they did get you off your butt in the short term, did they sustain your commitment in the long term?

Flogging ourselves for 'failure' is largely a waste of time. It saps our strength and vitality, and makes it hard to learn and grow from our experiences. A far more empowering response is 'self-acceptance' – which basically means letting go of all self-judgements.

Now before reading on, just pause for a ten-second 'check-in', and notice what your mind is saying.

★★★

Did your mind protest or argue? Did it leap up and down with joy? Did it point out all the flaws in my argument, or go along with it? Did it have a gripe about all these 'check-ins'? Did it tell you to skip the check-in, and carry on reading? Or did it go all quiet on you? All of these are perfectly normal reactions, so please thank your mind and carry on reading.

Let's return to the phrase 'letting go of all self-judgements'. When we make a mistake, or things go wrong, it's important to assess our *actions*; to reflect on what we did and what the results were. This is step 3 of the Confidence Cycle: 'assess the results'. We want to take a good, honest look at what we did, and assess it in terms of 'workability'. (Remember, workability refers to this question: Is what you are doing *working* to give you a rich and fulfilling life?) But this is very different to judging ourselves. Assessing our actions is workable. Judging ourselves is not.

Here's an example to draw out the difference.

Assessing my actions: 'When I got caught up in worrying about the shot, and lost my focus on the ball, I threw poorly and missed the basket.'

Judging myself: 'I am such a lousy basketball player.'

So self-acceptance does *not* mean that we pay no attention to the way we behave and the impact of our actions; it simply means we let go of blanket self-judgements. Why would we do this? Because judging ourselves does not help us in any way; it does not work to make our life richer and fuller.

Of course, knowing this intellectually won't stop it from happening. Our minds started judging us in early childhood; this pattern is not suddenly going to stop now. But what we *can* do is unhook ourselves from those self-judgements. And I invite you to start doing this, as of now.

Practise getting unhooked from *all* your self-judgements – both the negative *and* the positive. Let them float by like leaves on a stream. If your mind's telling you how crap you are, notice it and name it: *'Judgement.'* And if your mind's telling you how wonderful you are, notice it and name it: *'Judgement.'* (Remember, we don't want to hold on tightly to the positive *or* the negative self-judgements; we want to let go of them all.)

Also, feel free to be light-hearted with your naming. For example when you notice a positive self-judgement, you might playfully say to yourself, 'That's a lovely bit of flattery. Thanks mind.' And when you notice a negative one, you might say, 'Aha! The "I'm not good enough" story. Thanks mind!'

LET YOURSELF GO

Is a biography of Nelson Mandela the same thing as Nelson Mandela himself? Clearly not; it is nothing more than a construction of words and pictures. And regardless of how true or false those words are, and regardless of the quality of the photographs, they cannot come close to the richness and fullness of the living human being himself. (If you doubt this, then ask yourself: which would mean most to you – meeting your personal hero, or reading their biography?)

The same principle holds true for all your own self-judgements and self-descriptions; the biography of you is not you. Whether your mind describes you with glowing praise or sums you up with scathing criticism, the words it uses are nothing more than words. And you may recall, in ACT we're not too interested in whether those words are true or false; what we want to know is: are they helpful? If we allow these thoughts to guide our actions, will that work to make our lives richer and fuller?

Now if your mind is anything like mine, you'll notice your self-judgements change like the wind. Some days my mind tells me I'm a *wonderful* father, a *loving* husband and an *excellent* presenter; other days it tells me I'm a *lousy* father, a *selfish* husband and a *pathetic* presenter. There are days my mind says I'm a pretty good writer, and on other days it proclaims I write nothing but crap. The trick is, don't get attached to either story: the positive or the negative. Whether your mind says 'I'm wonderful' or 'I'm pathetic', 'I'm a winner' or 'I'm a loser', 'I'm successful' or 'I'm a failure', see it for what it is: just a story.

What matters most in life is what you do, what you stand for, the way you behave. This is far more important than the stories you believe about yourself. If you doubt this, think about your own funeral. Do you want people to be saying: 'What I really admired about him was that he was there for me when I needed him; he supported me; he encouraged me; he inspired me. He was a fantastic role model.' Or would you rather this: 'What I really admired about him was he had a very high opinion of himself'?

To quote the writer Margaret Fontey: 'One important thing I have learned over the years is the difference between taking one's work seriously and taking one's self seriously. The first is imperative, and the second is disastrous.'

POINTING THE FINGER

Most of us are far too quick to judge others: to label them as 'quitters', 'losers' or 'failures'. If we want to let go of judging ourselves harshly, we also need to do the same for others. The more we point the finger at our fellow human beings, and write them off as weak or inferior, the more we entrench the habit of harsh judgemental thinking. And sooner or later, our minds will turn those judgements back on ourselves.

Life is easier when we recognize there are no such people as 'quitters', 'losers' or 'failures'. There are just human beings, who – much like you and me – sometimes quit, sometimes lose and sometimes fail. Likewise, there are no such people as 'winners', 'champions' and 'successes'. Rather there are human beings who, just like you and me, sometimes win or are very successful in certain areas of their lives.

Tiger Woods provides a good example. For years he was idolized as a champion amongst champions: not only the world's top golfer, but the first athlete in history to earn more than a billion dollars. However, in November 2009, 'juicy' revelations about Tiger's long list of extramarital sexual partners dominated news headlines around the world. Thus, in terms of playing golf, he was highly successful; but in terms of building a trusting, respectful relationship with his wife, he failed miserably.

At this point, your mind may start protesting: 'Yes, but others succeed more than I do,' or 'I fail a lot more than others do.' If this happens, come back to the workability question: if you hold on tightly to those thoughts, will that help you to be who you want to be and do what you want to do?

I had to make this point to Michael, the businessman I mentioned earlier. Here's how the conversation went.

Michael: But it's true. I *am* a loser!

Russ: Michael, I am never going to get into a debate with you about whether your thoughts are true or not. I just want you to consider the situation. Your mind keeps calling you a loser, right?

Michael: Only about ten thousand times a day.

Russ: And I have to be honest with you; I don't know any way to stop your mind from doing that. This is what minds do. They are quick to judge us and criticize us.

Michael: Well, in my case it's justified.

Russ: Again, I'm not going to debate that with you. You've had lots of friends and business colleagues telling you that it wasn't your fault the company went down, and you don't need to be so harsh on yourself and so on, and that hasn't made any difference whatsoever has it? Your mind still tells you it's your fault, you're a loser, you screwed up.

Michael: Yes, because I did!

Russ: So here's the thing. If you hold on tightly to those thoughts, and get all caught up in them, does it help you? Does it help you to deal with the situation? To start over? To rebuild your life? Or does it just keep you feeling stuck and hopeless?

Michael: [Long pause] Stuck and hopeless.

Russ: So next time your mind starts judging you, what if you could let those thoughts come and go without getting all caught up in them? Would that be a useful ability?

Michael: [Long pause] Yes, it would.

I then took Michael through the techniques in this chapter, and I asked him to practise them regularly throughout the day. I specifically asked him to notice and name those thoughts – for example, 'Here's Radio Triple F again' or 'Aha! The good old "Loser" story.

Thanks mind!' – and let them come and go like leaves on a stream. When I saw Michael again, three weeks later, he reported that he'd been practising the techniques diligently, and he'd already developed a much greater sense of self-acceptance. He said that thoughts about being a loser were still showing up, but when they did, they hardly bothered him, and he usually found it quite easy to let them come and go. Michael's story reminds us: our self-judgements are not problematic in themselves – they only become so if we fuse with them.

Note: this is very different to repeating positive affirmations such as 'I completely accept myself.' Remember that self-esteem research I mentioned in chapter 3? It showed that when people with low self-esteem made affirmations of self-acceptance, they usually felt worse; it just got them thinking of all the things they *couldn't* truly accept about themselves.

This approach gives us yet another rule for the confidence game:

Rule 4: Self-acceptance trumps self-esteem.

THERE'S NO SHORTAGE OF HOOKS

We've looked at some of the mind's most common hooks: dwelling on obstacles, harsh self-judgements, comparisons to others, predictions of failure or disaster. But there are plenty of others: perfectionism, 'impostor syndrome' and rehashing old failures, to name but three.

Perfectionism results when we get bullied by thoughts such as: 'I have to do it perfectly', 'I mustn't make mistakes', 'I have to do it right first time' or 'If I can't do it well, there's no point in trying'. If we let these thoughts boss us around, it's a recipe for disaster. We become reluctant to try anything new for fear we won't do it well enough. Or we suffer from chronic stress, because we're always placing such high demands upon ourselves. Or we're continually disappointed or dissatisfied, because we don't live up to our own high expectations.

Impostor syndrome results when although you are skilled at what you're doing, you get hooked by thoughts that you're not competent: that you can't do it properly; that you've got away with it so far, but soon you'll be found out; that basically you're a fake, fraud or impostor. Naturally, if you buy into these thoughts, it will shake your confidence.

Yet another sure-fire way to undermine confidence is to replay and dwell on all our past failures. This readily leads to reason-giving: 'It's always gone badly in the past, there's no point trying again'; 'I failed the last two times, so why should this time be any different?' There are many other patterns of unhelpful thinking, but we don't need to list them all, because the principles are always the same: *If a thought has hooked you and pulled you away from living the life you want, then notice it, name it and neutralize it.*

At this point, you may be wondering, 'Okay, but what then? After I've unhooked myself, what do I do?' Excellent question.

chapter 8

the rules of engagement

Imagine listening to your favourite music with your ears full of cotton wool. Or watching your favourite movie wearing dark sunglasses. Or eating your favourite food while your tongue is still half-numb from a visit to the dentist. Or having a back massage while you're wearing a thick woollen jacket.

This is how we experience the world when we're all caught up in our thoughts. Remember the 'hands as thoughts' exercise from chapter 5? When your hands were covering your eyes (fusion), you were missing out on the world around you. But as you moved your hands away from your eyes (defusion), the world around you came into focus: you could see so much more clearly and 'take it all in'.

If we want to get the most out of life, we need to be fully present: aware, attentive and engaged in what is happening. This involves a mindfulness skill called 'engagement': connecting with the world through noticing what we can see, hear, touch, taste and smell.

The 'hands as thoughts' exercise demonstrates how defusion and engagement are related. As we defuse from our thoughts, we can connect and engage with the world, take more in and appreciate the present moment. Similarly, as we become 'present' and engage in the here-and-now, we spontaneously defuse from our thoughts. But what has all this to do with confidence?

THE POWER OF ENGAGEMENT

If you want to have great sex, or a great conversation, or a great game of golf; if you want to write well, sing well, run well; if you want to speak well, negotiate well or compete well, then you have to be *psychologically present*. You need to be *engaged* in what is happening.

Suppose you're playing tennis, and instead of keeping your attention on the ball, you focus on all the thoughts inside your head: 'Am I holding the racket correctly?', 'Are my feet in the best position?', 'Wow, that ball's coming so fast.' If your focus is on your thoughts rather than the ball, then what quality of game are you likely to play? Chances are, not very good. If you want to play well, you need to keep your attention on the ball.

Suppose you're making love, but instead of focusing on your partner, you're giving all your attention to thoughts in your head: 'How am I doing?', 'I can't hold on much longer', 'Is she really enjoying this?', 'What does he think of my body?' If you're all caught up in your thoughts, you won't find it a satisfying experience – especially if your mind is giving a running commentary on how you're performing. If you want to enjoy the experience, you need to be engaged in what you're doing: appreciating the pleasurable sensations, tuning in to your partner's responses, noticing the warmth and friction of your bodies, and letting your thoughts float past like clouds in the sky.

When you're in the heat of that important interview, sitting in front of the panel, you need to be engaged with the interviewers. You need to be 'tuned in' to what they are saying and how they're reacting. So the more attention you give to that commentary inside your head – 'D'oh! I shouldn't have said that', 'Oops, that didn't come out the way I wanted', 'Is this what they really want to hear?', 'Uh-oh, I don't like the expression on her face' – the harder you'll find it to focus, and the worse you'll perform.

In chapter 1, I mentioned Cleo, a shy twenty-eight-year-old scientist, who said that if she had more confidence, she would make more friends, socialize more and behave in a more genuine, warm and engaging way in social situations. Cleo told me that she found socializing quite stressful, and often closed down or clammed up. There were several contributing factors but the largest one was this: instead of paying attention to the person she was talking to, she would get caught up in thoughts like, 'I'm so boring', 'I don't know anything about this topic', 'I hope this person likes me' or 'I've got nothing to say.' And naturally, because she was so entangled in her thoughts, she found it hard to follow or contribute to the conversation, and didn't get much enjoyment out of it. Cleo had lost touch with the fact that if we want to socialize well, we need to pay attention to the other person: to notice what they are saying, their facial expressions and body language; to connect and engage with them.

When we say that someone looks confident, we have no idea what they are thinking or feeling. But we can observe what they are *doing;* how they are behaving. And one thing you'll always notice about confident people: they are very engaged in whatever they are doing. When they're socializing, they're thoroughly absorbed in the conversation. When they're playing sport, they're totally involved in the game. When they're writing a report, they're completely focused on the task. So whether we're talking about confidence the feeling *or* confidence the action, engagement always plays a major role.

Notice that in all the above scenarios, having negative thoughts is not the problem. The problem is that we are disengaged from our experiences. When we keep our attention on what we are doing and remain fully engaged in the task, then it doesn't matter what our minds say. Our thoughts only create problems if they hook us. If we let them come and go, then we can focus our attention on more important matters.

Now pause for twenty seconds, and notice what your mind is saying.

***

Is your mind enthusiastic and cooperative? Or is it just 'going with the flow'? Has it gone quiet on you? Or is it full of questions and objections? Here are a few concerns that often arise:

Q: Thinking is very useful. Surely you're not suggesting I let go of all my thoughts?

A: Not at all. If a thought is helpful – if it contains useful information that could help us to function better, perform better and build a better life, then it makes sense to use it; to let that thought influence our actions. However, in the examples above, the thoughts are clearly unhelpful, so it makes sense to let them come and go.

Q: But if I could just stop these negative thoughts from occurring in the first place, then there wouldn't be any problem, would there?

A: For sure. And I'm willing to bet you've already tried that. And it didn't work, did it? And if you want to try harder, be my guest. Just keep in mind that not even Zen masters, after a lifetime of mind training, develop the ability to eliminate negative thoughts.

Q: But when I'm in a challenging situation, it's hard to let my thoughts come and go. Isn't there an easier way?

A: Riding a bike, driving a car and using a pen all seem hard when we first start to learn them. Suppose I said to you, 'You know, learning to ride a bike at the age of forty-three is so hard. I've got no sense of balance, I'm wobbling all over the place, I'm afraid of falling off. I didn't know it would be so hard. I feel like giving up.' What would you say to me?

1. 'Yes, it's too hard, Russ. You might as well give up.'

2. 'Russ, there's no need for you to actually get on the bike and practise. Just go and read some books about bike-riding, and after that you should be able to ride well.'

3. 'Russ, of course it's hard initially, but if you keep getting on the bike and practising, then over time it'll get easier.'

Learning mindfulness skills is much the same as learning to ride a bike, play the piano or bake a cake. It may seem hard at the beginning, but it gets easier with practice. Fortunately, we can start learning mindfulness with simple, easy exercises. Indeed, some of the ones later in this chapter are almost effortless, and can be practised virtually any time, any place. This means we can progressively build up our skills, little by little, until we can be mindful even in the most challenging situations. (Note: I assume you've been doing the exercises in previous chapters. If not, please go back and work through them, as they provide a foundation for the work that follows shortly.) We'll now talk a little more about the theory of engagement, and then we'll knuckle down to actually doing it.

DON'T JUST DO SOMETHING: BE THERE!

Time for a quick refresher. The golden rule of the confidence game is this:

The actions of confidence come first; the feelings of confidence come later.

Only when we can *do* something well are we likely to *feel* confident. But it is almost impossible to do something well if we are not engaged in what we are doing. If we 'just do it' mindlessly, lost in our thoughts, or we go through the motions on automatic pilot, then we probably won't do it very well.

So how do we engage in our experiences? Simple. We pay attention. We notice what is happening, here and now. Paying attention is at the very core of mindfulness. But it's not just paying attention in any old way. Mindfulness means paying attention with openness, curiosity and flexibility. Let's break that down.

Paying attention: we pay attention to what is happening in this moment, in both our 'inner world' and the world outside us. In other words, we notice what we're thinking and feeling, and also what we can see, hear, touch, taste and smell.

Openness: we are open to what is happening, even if we don't like or approve of it, as opposed to turning away or closing off from our experiences.

Curiosity: we are curious about what is happening. We actively seek to discover something new in our experience; something we may have missed, or taken for granted. Like an intrepid explorer or an enthusiastic scientist, we pay attention to the details, taking nothing for granted, interested in whatever we may find.

Flexibility: we are flexible in the way we pay attention. At times we may have a narrow focus, such as when we are absorbed in a task: threading a needle, drilling a hole or hitting a golf ball. At other times we may have a broad focus, such as when we are exploring a new city and taking in all the novel sights, smells and sounds. At times we may be more focused on the inner world of our thoughts and feelings. And at other times we may focus more on the external world.

So how about we try this out right now? I invite you to stop reading for a few moments and simply notice what you can hear. Notice the sounds coming from yourself – your breathing and your movements. Then expand your awareness to notice the sounds around you. Listen to these sounds as if you were a musician appreciating great music: notice the different pitches, volumes and rhythms; notice how some sounds fade or cease, while others start or grow louder. Please do this now for thirty seconds.

★★★

Next, I invite you to look around and notice five things you can see. Look at each object as if you were an artist studying a famous masterpiece. Notice the shape, colour, texture and shading; notice any shadows, reflections or highlights. Take thirty to sixty seconds to do this, lingering with curiosity on each object – no matter how familiar or mundane it seems.

★★★

Now sit up straight in your chair and notice the position of your body. Push your feet firmly into the floor, straighten your spine and drop your shoulders. Take thirty seconds to scan your body from head to toe, noticing what you can feel in each part of it. Do this with intense curiosity, as if you were a scientist from another planet who has been granted the experience of thirty seconds inside a human body.

★★★

Now do all of the above simultaneously. Put the book down, sit up straight, plant your feet firmly, and flexibly focus your attention: from your body, to what you can see, to what you can hear. Please do this now for thirty seconds.

★★★

So what happened? Did you become more 'present': more aware of your surroundings and your body? When we're lost in a book, we lose touch with almost everything except those words on the page in front of us. However, those words are only one small aspect of our experience in the present moment. When we put the book down and pay attention to our bodies and our environment, we become aware of all sorts of sights, sounds and sensations.

Now getting lost in a book is not a bad thing. Indeed, it's one of my favourite pastimes. But what if you were permanently lost in a book? Suppose that all day long, you were walking around with your head literally buried in a book; holding it in your hands and reading it avidly at the same time as you were eating dinner, playing with your kids, making love, driving your car, playing tennis or making conversation. How would that affect your life, health and relationships?

We all have a natural tendency to lead our lives in this manner. The only difference is, instead of being lost in a book, we are lost in all those words inside our head. Engagement means that in much the same way as we can put down a book, we let go of the words inside our head and pay attention to other aspects of our experience.

THE STAGE SHOW OF LIFE

Life is like a magnificent stage show. And on that stage are all our emotions, memories, images, thoughts and sensations, as well as everything we can see, hear, touch, taste and smell. Mindfulness is like the lighting system: we can bring up the lights on any part of the show at any time so we can see all the details. The lighting doesn't alter what happens on the stage, but it affects how we perceive and appreciate the show.

We have a lot of flexibility with this lighting system. We can dim the lights and shine spotlights on key areas of action – or we can bring up all the lights simultaneously, and watch the entire show at once.

The 'leaves on a stream' exercise is like dimming the lights on the stage and shining a spotlight on your thoughts. And in the brief exercises you did a few moments ago, you played around with the spotlights, illuminating various aspects of the show: what you could see, what you could hear, and what you could feel.

So, given that there are so many different aspects to the stage show, what should we focus on? The answer is simple. Focus on whatever is most important in this moment; pay attention to whatever helps us be the person we want to be, and do the things we want to do.

Psychologists often refer to this as 'task-focused attention': being fully focused on the task at hand. If we want to perform any task well – whether it's golfing, painting, driving, making love, making lunch or making conversation – our attention needs to be centred on whatever is relevant to the task. Negative self-judgements, predictions of failure, thoughts about not being good enough: these are not relevant parts of the stage show. But we can't get them off the stage, and nor can we plunge them into absolute darkness. So what can we do? We can dim the lights a little on those areas, and focus the bright spotlights where they're needed: on the lead singer, the musicians, or the dancers, rather than on the roadies and the security guards. The exercise that follows will show you how.

MINDFUL BREATHING

The practice of mindful breathing is thousands of years old. You can find it in religious, spiritual and philosophical traditions as diverse as Hinduism, Judaism, Taoism, Buddhism, Christianity, Islam, yoga, tai chi and many martial arts. It's a simple but effective way to develop engagement and defusion skills, and you can do it for as long as you like, from thirty seconds to thirty minutes. If you've never done anything like this before, I recommend you start with just five minutes. Over time, you can increase the duration.

(A note of caution: if you have a longstanding habit of shallow, rapid breathing, then the slow, deep breathing of this exercise may at first seem odd or uncomfortable. However, if you persist with it, then within a couple of weeks of daily practice it will start to feel natural and comfortable. Also, it's very uncommon, but mindful breathing can occasionally bring up feelings of anxiety or dizziness for some people. If this happens to you, I strongly encourage you to persist (I guarantee you won't pass out, even if your mind tells you that you will); and within a week or two, such reactions usually disappear.

Now please read the instructions twice, so you know what you're doing, and then give it a go. (And if you'd like a voice to guide you through it, I've recorded this exercise on *Mindfulness Skills: Volume 1*, available as a CD or MP3 from www.thehappiness trap.co.uk.)

- Find a comfortable position (preferably seated upright, with your back straight, and your feet flat on the ground).
- Close your eyes or fix on a spot, whichever you prefer.
- Take some gentle, slow, deep breaths.
- Focus on emptying your lungs. Gently and calmly push out every last bit of air, until your lungs are completely empty, and then allow them to fill by themselves.
- There's no need to take a deep breath in; once your lungs are empty, they will automatically refill. See if you can simply *allow* this to happen, rather than forcing it.
- Observe your breathing as if you are a curious scientist who has never encountered anything like it before. Notice every little sensation: the air moving in and out of your nostrils; the rise and fall of your shoulders; the lifting and lowering of your ribcage; the rise and fall of your abdomen. Notice how all these elements interact effortlessly.
- After the first ten breaths, allow your breathing to find its own natural rhythm. There's no need to keep controlling it.
- Your challenge is to keep the spotlight on your breath; to observe it flowing in and out of your body. As you do this, let your thoughts float by like leaves on a stream.
- From time to time, your mind will hook you and pull you out of the exercise. You'll get caught up in everything and anything, from ancient memories to daydreams to what you're having for dinner. This is natural and normal, and it will keep on happening. Each time you realize you've been hooked, gently acknowledge it and refocus on your breath. (And if your mind starts to beat you up for not doing it well enough, thank it for those thoughts and carry on with the exercise.)

119

- If uncomfortable feelings show up, such as frustration, boredom, impatience, anxiety or backache, silently acknowledge them. Say to yourself, 'Here's boredom' or 'Here's frustration.' Then refocus on your breath.

- Periodically your mind is likely to grumble or protest: 'I can't do it', 'It's too hard', 'It's boring.' At first, these thoughts – and many others – will hook you and pull you out of the exercise. But they are really not a problem. No matter how many hundreds or thousands of times your mind hooks you, as soon as you realize it, acknowledge it, unhook and refocus on the breath. Every time you do this, you are building a valuable skill: the ability to sustain focus.

- Once your time is up, expand your awareness to engage with the world around you. Keeping a spotlight on your breath, also bring up the lights on your body and your environment: push your feet into the floor, sit up straight, have a good stretch and notice what can you see, hear, touch, taste and smell.

Once you have read the instructions at least twice, please do the exercise. Five minutes is a good length of time to begin with, but you can do more or less than that if you prefer.

DID YOU GET HOOKED?

How did you go with the exercise? If you've never done anything like this before, you are doing well if you last even ten seconds before you get hooked and pulled out of it. When we are new to mindfulness, most of us are shocked at just how hard it is to stay focused. Of course, most of us have discovered certain activities in which we *can* maintain focus for long periods. These might include: watching movies, reading books, having great conversations, or participating in a sport, hobby or creative pursuit. But once you step outside of your comfort zone, and try to focus in more challenging situations – for example, when you're learning a difficult skill or trying to meet a tight deadline, or you have to attend a meeting with somebody difficult – then you will usually find it much harder.

So, mindful breathing is an excellent way to improve your ability to focus. And naturally, the more you practise, the better you'll get. (Does that last sentence give you a sense of déjà vu?)

The exercise above is mindful breathing in its most basic, 'no-frills' form. However, there are various elements that you can add to the exercise that might make it easier or more interesting. I invite you to try them out the next few times you practise, and find out which approach works best for you.

Option 1: Counting the breath

Count each breath you take, silently saying the number as you exhale. Once you reach ten, go back down to one and start again. If at any point you lose track of the numbers, simply start again from one.

Option 2: Coloured breath

Visualize the breath flowing into and out of your lungs, as if it were coloured. You can imagine your breath any colour you like; most people choose white.

Option 3: White light and dark clouds

You can imagine yourself breathing in white light as you inhale, and breathing out dark clouds as you exhale.

Option 4: Repeating words

You can silently repeat words as you breathe in and out. For example, you can slowly say, 'Breathing in' as you inhale and 'Breathing out' as you exhale. Or you might simply say, 'In' and 'Out'.

Option 5: Balloon breathing

You can imagine a balloon inside your abdomen that gradually expands as you breathe in, and deflates as you breathe out.

Any Time, Any Place

One of the great things about mindful breathing is we can practise it any time, any place. I encourage you to practise it at:

- Red traffic lights
- Waiting in queues
- During commercial breaks on TV
- Sitting on the toilet
- When you arrive early for a meeting, interview or social event
- In bed as you drift off to sleep or wake up
- When you're on hold on the telephone
- Whenever you have time to kill: as you wait for a bus, train or aeroplane, or for your partner to get ready, or for a movie to begin

On top of all these informal mini-exercises, I encourage you to create a schedule for formal practice. For example, in the first week you might set aside five minutes two or three times a day to sit somewhere quietly and practise mindful breathing. You might then increase the duration by thirty seconds each day, until by week three you are doing this for ten minutes two or three times a day.

Keep in mind that every little bit of practice counts. Even one minute a day is better than none at all. To help develop the habit you could use some simple reminders. Why not stick a label on your fridge or your car dashboard that says 'Breathe', 'Engage' or 'Practise'? You could also use your computer or mobile phone: set a reminder to pop up in your calendar each day. Another option is to put a brightly coloured sticker on the strap of your watch, or on your wallet or purse; this way, whenever you check the time or open your wallet or purse, you notice the sticker and it reminds you to take a few mindful breaths.

You could also plan in advance: if you know there's a good chance you'll be stuck waiting somewhere, such as when attending a doctor's appointment, or catching a plane, then make a commitment before you get there that you'll spend at least some of that time mindfully breathing.

BREATHING IS JUST THE START

Mindful breathing is a useful practice in its own right. It allows us to take some time out from our busy daily routines, and often creates a restful state that allows us to recharge our batteries and find some inner peace. However, I'd like you to think of it as a versatile training tool to help you engage fully in every meaningful task in your life. When you're playing sport, working out, writing that book, making that sculpture, painting that canvas, playing that instrument, making love, playing with your kids, dancing at a party, making conversation, giving that speech or negotiating that deal, instead of shining the spotlight on your breath, shine it on the task that you are doing; engage fully in the experience and let your thoughts come and go like passing cars.

And what if you don't like mindful breathing? Well, I encourage you to practise it anyway, because even if you don't like it at first, most people find as time goes on it gets easier and more rewarding. However, if you're absolutely opposed to it, there are many other ways of developing engagement skills. All you need do is to stop and . . .

chapter 9

smell the roses

It is a twenty-minute march from your cramped, gloomy prison cell to the limestone quarry. Once there, you will slave away with your pick and shovel under the searing sun, your hands blistered and bleeding, your body drenched with sweat and plastered with dust.

How would you feel if you were on that march, knowing what lay in store for you? In his autobiography, *Long Walk to Freedom,* Nelson Mandela described this march as a 'tonic'. For thirteen of his years in Robben Island prison, he did it every single morning. And as he did so, he engaged fully in his experience: he noticed the birds flying gracefully through the sky, the cool caress of the wind blowing in from the sea and the fresh smell of the eucalyptus blossoms. He wasn't lost in thoughts about the hard work ahead of him or the miserable days behind him; he was living fully in the present moment.

Fortunately, we don't have to be locked away in prison to appreciate the birds, the wind and the flowers. If we stop rushing around on automatic pilot and use our five senses to connect fully with the world around us, we will find much more fulfilment. Yes, we all know the saying, 'Stop and smell the roses', but how often do we actually do it?

The exercises in this chapter all involve engaging through the five senses: noticing what you can see, hear, touch, taste and smell. This is to help you develop your ability to stay present, focused and absorbed in whatever you are doing. As we have discussed, this ability is essential if you want to do anything well, or find it satisfying.

MINDFULNESS FOR BUSY PEOPLE

I have occasionally met people who had 'too much time on their hands', but I have to say, they are few and far between. Most of us are busy, busy, busy. Many of my clients tell me they 'don't have time to practise all this stuff'. Indeed, I often have the same thoughts myself. But the beauty of mindfulness training is that you can do it any time, any place. Sure, if you're going to sit and do a formal exercise such as ten minutes of mindful breathing or ten minutes of 'leaves on a stream', you'll need to make some time for that. (And I strongly encourage you to do so!) But throughout the day, there are all sorts of opportunities for practice without having to alter your daily routine. Here are a few suggestions.

ENGAGING IN YOUR MORNING ROUTINE

You can turn any part of your morning routine into a mindfulness training session: brushing your teeth, shaving, going to the toilet, having a shower, getting dressed, making the bed, making breakfast, eating breakfast, having a cup of tea, etc. Specifically practise developing your engagement and defusion skills. For example, if you're making a cup of tea, engage in every little step of the process, using all five senses. And observe what is happening with the utmost curiosity, as if you've never done it before.

Notice all the different sounds involved, listening to the changes in pitch, volume, timbre and rhythm: the crescendo of the kettle filling up, the sharp click of the 'on' switch, the rumble of boiling water, the hiss of escaping steam, the 'swoosh' as you pour the water into the cup, the trickle as you lift the teabag out, and the gentle 'splosh' as you add sugar or milk.

Notice all the different visual elements, including shapes, colours, textures, and light and shadow: the thick rush of steam spouting from the kettle; the misty swirls of steam rising from the water in the cup; the light rippling on the surface as you dunk the teabag; the dark stream of tea diffusing through the hot water; the fluffy clouds of milk billowing up to the surface.

Notice all the different body movements required: the effortless interaction of your shoulder, arm, hand and eyes as you're lifting up the kettle, turning on the tap, replacing the kettle, pouring the water, dunking the teabag and so on.

As you do this, see if you can discover something new: something you previously took for granted. Have you ever *truly* paid attention to the patterns of steam rising from your cup, or the sound of the spoon clinking against the side, or the movement of your shoulder when you dunk a teabag?

As you do this practice, your mind will try to hook you with thoughts about all the things on your to-do list. Let those thoughts come and go like passing cars, and engage in what you are doing here and now. Of course, from time to time your mind will pull you out of it. The moment you realize this, gently acknowledge it, unhook yourself, and engage once again in making the tea.

ENGAGING IN A CHORE

Are there any dull, tedious or mundane chores in your life; things that you just have to do to make your life work? Do you grit your teeth and rush through them as quickly as possible? Or do you do them mindlessly, going through the motions on automatic pilot? Or do you try to make them less boring by listening to the radio or watching TV simultaneously?

Common examples might include ironing clothes, doing the washing-up, stacking the dishwasher, putting out the rubbish, making lunch for the kids, vacuuming, doing the laundry, sweeping the floor, scrubbing the bathtub and so on. Any of these chores provide valuable opportunities to develop engagement and defusion skills.

Remember Seb, the taxi driver afraid to make love to his wife? Seb recognized that if he ever wanted to enjoy sexual activity again, he would have to learn how to engage fully in the process, instead of getting lost in his anxious thoughts and feelings. So he chose to turn stacking the dishwasher into a mindfulness practice. I said to him, 'Next time you have to stack the dishwasher, imagine you are the world champion of dishwasher-stackers, and your performance is being filmed and beamed live to hundreds of millions of TV sets around the world.' I asked him to place in every single cup, plate, bowl, spoon, knife and fork with the greatest of care. To put each item down gently, noticing the sound it made as it slotted into place. To notice the colours and patterns that food and drink have left on its surface. To notice the movements of his shoulder, arm and hand. And I reminded him, 'As you do this, let your mind chatter away like a radio in the background. And whenever you get hooked, acknowledge it, unhook and refocus.'

At our next session Seb reported that he had tried this approach, and much to his surprise, stacking the dishwasher had turned into an engaging activity rather than a task of mindless drudgery. 'Don't get me wrong,' he said. 'It's not like it's turned into fun. If I had a choice between watching football and stacking the dishwasher, believe me, football would win hands down. But it's different when I do it mindfully. I kind of get absorbed in it.

It's weird; it's kind of interesting. I didn't think stacking dishes could be interesting.'

ENGAGING IN A PLEASURABLE ACTIVITY

Each and every day, we do many things that are potentially very pleasurable, but we fail to maximize the enjoyment and satisfaction of these experiences because we're not fully engaged. We take them for granted, or do them on autopilot while thinking about what we have to do next. Common examples include: eating, drinking, playing with your kids, stroking a pet, having a shower, or hugging a loved one.

We also miss out on many simple pleasures purely because we're too busy to 'stop and smell the roses'. What could you do, simply and easily, that could add some pleasure to your life? Could you go for a walk in the park and appreciate the birds and the flowers? Could you listen to more of your favourite music? Could you cook something special? Could you add a bit of spice to your sex life?

Each day, I invite you to practise mindfulness of at least two pleasurable experiences. If you're having a shower, use all five senses to engage in it: notice the patterns of the droplets on the shower screen, the sensations of the water on your skin, the smell of the shampoo and soap, and the sound of the spray coming out of the nozzle.

When you're eating dinner, pause for a moment before your first bite, and notice the different aromas of the various ingredients, and the colours, shapes and textures of the different foods. Then, as you cut up the food, notice the sounds made by your cutlery and the movements of your hands and arms and shoulders. And as you eat that first mouthful, notice the tastes and textures in your mouth, as if you were a gourmet food critic who has never tasted a meal like this before.

If you're hugging someone you love, notice the sensations in your body, and the way you position yourself, and what you do with your arms, and the reactions in the face and body of your loved one.

ENGAGING IN ANYTHING AND EVERYTHING

As you can see, there are countless 'quick and easy' ways for busy people to develop mindfulness. And remember, you can put literally anything 'in the spotlight' and practise sustaining your focus on it: from tying your shoelaces to blowing your nose; from watching a sunset to washing your hair; from mowing the lawn to scratching your backside (not that *you'd* ever do that, of course!).

So invent a few engagement practices of your own: from mindfully stocking the fridge to mindfully walking up the stairs; from mindfully combing your hair to mindfully unlocking the front door. Remember, every mindful moment makes a difference. The more practice we do, the less we'll wander off into . . .

chapter 10

psychological smog

I could hardly believe my eyes. I was walking through the botanic gardens in Melbourne, but I could have been just about anywhere. A few minutes earlier, I had been surrounded by magnificent trees. Presumably the trees hadn't moved, but now I could not see the slightest trace of them. The smog had obliterated everything.

Melbourne is a beautiful city and fortunately it very rarely suffers from smog attacks, but when it happens, it's dramatic. And if you've ever been caught in smog, fog, torrential rain, a blizzard or a dust storm, then you'll know how frustrating it is; it's hard to get where you're going when you can't see clearly. Still, at least when we're trapped by the weather, we *know* it's happening, and we can modify our behaviour as required. But when we get trapped inside our 'psychological smog', it's a different story.

Psychological smog is what it sounds like: a thick cloud of thoughts which prevents us from seeing clearly or acting effectively. And sadly, most of the time, when we are lost in this smog, we don't even realize it. It's only once the smog lifts and we reconnect with the world and start to see clearly that we recognize how lost we really were.

Psychological smog takes many forms: worrying, blaming, fantasizing, rehashing old rejections and failures, planning escapes, plotting revenge, daydreaming, rehearsing conversations, 'analysis paralysis', dwelling on times long gone and predicting the future. And if we're not mindful, we can spend hours wandering fruitlessly through this smog, all the while missing out on our lives.

But there's one thing we need to be clear on:

The smog is not created by our thoughts. It is fusion with our thoughts that creates the smog.

In other words, no matter how negative, unhelpful or painful our thoughts might be, they will *not* create smog if we are defused from them. But the more we fuse with them, the thicker the smog, and the more we lose contact with the world around us. The only way out of the smog is through engagement and defusion. The instant we unhook ourselves from those thoughts and engage fully in whatever we are doing, we can see clearly and take effective action.

THE WORRY SMOG

One of the most suffocating forms of psychological smog is worrying. We all worry to some degree, but the more habitual it becomes, the more it drains our vitality. It wastes time, saps energy, and gets in the way of effective action. All the clients I've mentioned so far wasted plenty of time worrying. Raj worried endlessly about the possibility of losing money with his new restaurant venture. Seb worried about whether he would ever be able to have 'good sex' again, and whether or not his wife would leave him if he didn't 'satisfy' her. Sarah worried about screwing up her auditions. And Cleo and Claire both worried a lot about being rejected, or clamming up in social situations.

All of these people reduced their worrying significantly using the techniques in this chapter. But at no point did I say to them 'Stop worrying about it.' In my opinion, that's one of the most useless bits of advice you could possibly give someone. After all, if it were that easy to stop, they probably would have done so long before we so wisely suggested it.

In fact, many of my clients complain: 'I try to stop worrying, but I can't.' Comments like this don't surprise me. There's a lot of research now which shows that trying to stop worrying usually just makes it worse; when we 'push away' worrying thoughts or distract ourselves from them, it often gives us some short-term relief, but in the long term it generally leads to a rebound effect, where those thoughts return with greater frequency and intensity than before. So how then do we deal with the 'worry smog'?

Step 1: Be clear about what 'worrying' is
Worrying does not mean having thoughts about 'bad' things that might happen. We all have such thoughts, and as with any other form of psychological smog, the thoughts themselves are not the problem; the problem is *fusion*. Worrying means *fusing* with those thoughts: holding on tightly to them, replaying them over and over instead of letting them go.

Step 2: Identify the costs of worrying
The major cost of worrying is missing out on life. When we're all caught up in our worries, we are not 'psychologically present'. We are disconnected from our here-and-now experiences, and are instead caught up in thoughts about the future. We miss out on interaction with our loved ones; we miss out on the food we are

eating or the activities we are doing; we go through the motions, but we are not present, and so the experience is not rewarding or fulfilling. And it certainly interferes with our performance, in any field of endeavour. (Note: fear and anxiety do *not* interfere with performance, but worrying does.) Other costs include wasted time, disrupted sleep and procrastination over important decisions.

Step 3: Unhook from reasons to worry

Sometimes my clients say to me: 'That's just me. I've always been a worrier. I can't help it.' I usually reply: 'If you go along with that story, where does it leave you? It's quite natural that your mind would say something like that. Our minds tend to get very set in their ways, and they often don't like making changes. So how about we let your mind say that change is impossible, and let's give it a go anyway and see what happens?'

Another classic story I often hear is this: 'But worrying helps me.' The story usually goes that worrying is helpful for 'dealing with my problems' or 'preparing for the worst'. I reply that worrying is like riding a rickety old bicycle. It will get you from A to B, but how long will it take you, and what condition will you be in by the time you get there? There are far more effective ways to make this journey: with an excellent new bicycle, or by car, bus or plane.

If we want to *effectively* solve our problems, or *effectively* make decisions for the future, or *effectively* prepare for action in the event of worst-case scenarios, then worrying simply does not do the job. It typically impairs action, increases procrastination, reduces motivation and leads to poor decision-making, while increasing stress and anxiety.

Instead of worrying, move to active planning or constructive problem-solving using questions like these:

What can I do to deal effectively with this situation? What action could I take that might make a difference? Where could I get help or advice?

What's the worst thing that could happen? If it did happen, what could I do to cope? What actions could I take, or help/advice could I get?

If you can take effective action, do so. If you can't, then make room for your discomfort, defuse from your worries, and engage in doing something meaningful, here and now.

Step 4: Distinguish worrying from taking care

Many people seem to think that worrying about their problems equates to taking care of their problems. But there is a huge difference: the former is useless, the latter invaluable.

Worrying about your health: uselessly dwelling on scary stories about what might be wrong with your body.

Taking care of your health: eating well, exercising, stopping smoking.

Worrying about your finances: uselessly dwelling on scary stories about how little money you have, or how you might lose it, or what you may be unable to afford.

Taking care of your finances: starting a savings account, setting a budget, meeting with a financial adviser.

Step 5: Defuse from worrying itself

Our mind is like the world's greatest storyteller, and all it wants is our attention. And it knows that we pay attention when it tells us scary stories. So it's not going to suddenly stop doing that. But we can learn to let those worries come and go, without buying into them. One simple technique is to notice and name: as soon as we become aware of worrying thoughts, we silently say to ourselves: 'Here's worrying again!' or more simply, 'Worrying'. And if it's worrying about a recurrent theme, you might also try Thanking Your Mind and/or Naming the Story: 'Aha! Here's the "Going bankrupt" story! Thanks Mind!' or 'Aha! Here's the "Lose the race" story! Thanks Mind!' Also, regular practice of 'leaves on a stream' or mindful breathing is extremely useful for chronic worriers.

FROM SMOG TO CONFIDENCE

Any mindfulness technique is helpful for escaping from *any* form of psychological smog. In the previous chapter, I talked about simple ways of developing mindfulness skills in everyday life. We're now going to tie all this in to your major life goals. First, a quick revisit of the Confidence Cycle:

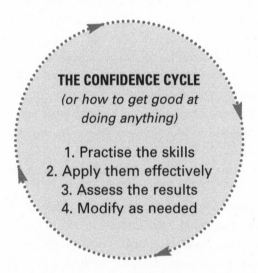

THE CONFIDENCE CYCLE
(or how to get good at doing anything)

1. Practise the skills
2. Apply them effectively
3. Assess the results
4. Modify as needed

Consider for a moment: in which fields of endeavour would genuine confidence make the most difference to you: sports, business, social, creative or something else? I invite you now to choose one of these fields, whichever one you'd like to focus on first, and think about it in terms of the Confidence Cycle. To improve what you do in this field, what skills will you need to actively work on?

For example, in sport you might need to practise a particular technique, manoeuvre or movement, such as a golf swing or a tennis serve. In business, you may need to practise your presentation skills, interview technique or sales pitch. In socializing, you may need to practise telling jokes or stories, asking open-ended questions, or sharing more of yourself. In painting, you may need to practise mixing pigments, drawing up perspective grids or experimenting with light and shadow. In parenting, you may need to practise giving positive feedback, being assertive or engaging your kids on their level.

Often we are reluctant to accept the need for practice, but there's really no escaping it. Our minds may protest: *'But it's not fair. Some people are naturally talented. They don't have to do all this practice. Why should I?'* I have no doubt that such thoughts are true. All humans are *not* born equal, and some are naturally talented in certain areas. We can see this even in young children: some are naturally stronger, faster, more coordinated, more imaginative, better with words and so on than their peers. The important question is this: if we hold on tightly to this thought, will it help us do what we need to do to improve – or will it just set us up for frustration and resentment?

I must admit, I often feel envious when others get better results than me with (apparently) less effort – such as novelist Iain Banks, who writes one book each year, and it only takes him three months to do it! However, I usually unhook myself quickly from the 'It's not fair' story, as I recognise holding on to it doesn't help me. (That doesn't get rid of my envy, but it does help me to get out of the smog.)

I also find it helpful to remember this: very often those people who seem 'naturally talented' have *already done* a lot more practice than we have to get to where they are. For example, Tiger Woods started playing golf at the age of two and Mozart started playing the keyboard at the age of four. Sure, they had natural talent compared to other kids their age, but by the time they started showing phenomenal results in adulthood, they had put in an astonishing amount of practice.

For a more down-to-earth example, consider those folks who are socially very confident. These people, the life blood of every social event, were not born with the so-called 'gift of the gab'. Like you and me, they were born unable to speak, and it took plenty of practice to get where they are. Of course, most of them didn't consciously decide, 'I'm going to go and practise my conversational skills'; more than likely, they developed their skills spontaneously through doing what gave them fulfilment. And while they may well have had a 'natural talent' for social interaction, this doesn't alter the fact that improvement requires practice.

So if you want to get good at making conversation, but you 'can never think of anything interesting to say' and you're 'not much of a storyteller', then you're going to have to practise telling anecdotes in an engaging manner. If you want to get good at writing thrillers, then you'll need to practise developing plots and characters, writing snappy dialogue, and setting up tension and conflict. If you want to serve well in tennis . . . well, you get the picture. I could fill a whole book with variants on this sentence, but it'd get a bit tedious, so why not fill in the blanks for yourself:

If I want to get good at _____ *then I'll need to practise* _____

Once you've identified an important skill to practise, the next step — you guessed it — is to do it mindfully. In other words, specifically turn this practice into an opportunity to develop defusion and engagement. If you're stretching before a training session, do those stretches mindfully. If you're rehearsing your answers for an interview, say them mindfully. If you're doing a warm-up on your instrument, play those scales mindfully. There are at least three significant benefits from doing this.

The first big benefit is that mindfulness is the antidote to boredom. A common reason we give for not practising is that 'It's boring.' However, if we are experiencing boredom, that means we have disengaged from what we are doing; instead we have fused with a story that the activity is dull or tedious, and there are other, far more interesting things that we could be doing.

But if we unhook ourselves from this story and engage fully in the activity, there is no boredom. Boredom and mindfulness can't occur simultaneously: mindfulness involves *paying attention* to what is happening with openness and *curiosity*; boredom involves *inattention* to what is happening, and a *lack* of curiosity.

So to enhance your ability to engage, cultivate curiosity about what you are doing. Even if you've done it a million times before, no two sessions are ever identical; what can you notice that's different, or that you've previously taken for granted?

The second big benefit is that whatever skill you practise, you will get much better results if you do it mindfully than if you go through the motions on autopilot. Remember, step 2 of the Confidence Cycle is *applying skills effectively*; this is not possible unless we pay attention to what we are doing. If we want to play tennis well, then we 'spotlight' the tennis ball. If we want to drive a car well, we 'spotlight' the road and the traffic. If we want to socialize well, we 'spotlight' the words and body language of the other person.

The third big benefit is that this approach paves the way for peak performance. If you want to perform at your best in any given role – in business, or as a parent, partner, athlete, performer, artist or lover – then you'll not only need to have good skills, but the ability to remain focused on and engaged in what you're doing.

So make a commitment now:

- What essential skills will you start practising mindfully?
- How much will you practise them: specify when, where and for how long?

And please don't take my word about the benefits; try it for yourself and see the difference it makes.

WHAT IF MY SKILLS ARE GOOD ENOUGH?

There may well be no problem with your skill levels. For example, research shows that most people with significant social anxiety do not actually lack social skills; they're just fused with stories about being dull, boring or unlikeable, or saying something stupid, boring or unfunny. Similarly, people who suffer from 'impostor syndrome' have no actual deficit in their skills; they are just fused with the story that they're a fake, fraud or impostor. However, even if this is the case, there's always room for improving important skills. As Tiger Woods puts it: 'No matter how good you get, you can always get better – and that's the exciting part.' So please do choose at least one important skill and commit to doing it mindfully, as suggested above.

HOW MUCH MINDFULNESS ARE YOU PRACTISING?

Here's my prediction: by this point in the book, many readers will be enthusiastically practising their mindfulness skills and reaping the rewards. Many others will be reading the book but *not* actually practising the exercises because they're repeatedly getting hooked by thoughts such as, 'It's all too hard', 'I'll start it later', 'I don't have the energy', 'I can't be bothered', 'I shouldn't have to do this' and a myriad of other forms of reason-giving. Therefore, in the next section of the book, we're going to look at self-motivation, an essential skill for winning the game of confidence.

part three

what gets you going?

chapter 11

fuelling up

'During my lifetime I have dedicated myself to this struggle of the African people. I have fought against white domination and I have fought against black domination. I have cherished the ideal of a democratic and free society in which all persons live together in harmony and with equal opportunities. It is an ideal which I hope to live for and to achieve. But if needs be, it is an ideal for which I am prepared to die.' *Nelson Mandela*

The above quote is Mandela's closing statement from the infamous Rivonia trial. The South African government had high expectations for the trial: they wanted to impose the death sentence on Mandela and other leaders of the democracy movement. However, due to international protests and sanctions against South Africa, they relented and imposed harsh prison sentences instead.

Mandela's values come shining through in his speech: democracy, freedom, equality and cooperation. Those values kept him going through thick and thin: through establishing a legal firm to provide free or low-cost legal support for poor black people; through the many years he spent underground, hiding from the police while inciting non-violent resistance against the government; throughout his twenty-seven gruelling years of imprisonment; and during his term as the first democratically elected president of South Africa. And any time he felt frightened, demoralized or exhausted, those values gave him the strength to persevere.

In prison, Mandela realized that the government could take away his freedom, but they couldn't take away his values. He believed that good education was essential for democracy and equality, and he was determined to make it available for one and all. So he established an underground 'university': prisoners would secretly meet in the mineshafts to discuss ideas, share knowledge, attend lectures and teach each other everything from politics to Shakespeare. (Later this became known as 'Nelson Mandela University'.)

He also studied Afrikaans, the language of white South Africans, and took every opportunity to discuss South African politics and history with the white warders. This gave him great insight into the attitudes and belief systems of the white Boer minority, which later became invaluable when he had to negotiate a new South African constitution. And in his later years in prison, when his conditions were a bit better, he even completed a law degree by correspondence.

So what has all this to do with confidence? To answer that question, we need to revisit values and goals.

VALUES AND GOALS REVISITED

Most books and courses on self-development place a major focus on goal-setting. Especially when they cover topics such as confidence, success and peak performance. And rightly so, because

144

goals are important. However, if we want the best chance of achieving our goals, we'd do well to clarify our values first. Why? For at least three reasons.

1. Values give us the inspiration and motivation to persist; to do what needs to be done, even when the going gets rough.

If our goals are a long way off, or very difficult, or there are major obstacles in the way, then without values to keep us motivated, we'll often run out of steam before we get there. Mandela's values sustained him throughout a lifetime of fear, anguish and heartbreak: without them, he would never have achieved what he did.

2. Values give us guidance.

Values are like a compass: they guide our journeys, give us direction and keep us on track. If we pursue goals that are not aligned with our core values, it almost always leads to disappointment and dissatisfaction. But if we use our values to set personally meaningful goals, the opposite holds true.

3. Values provide us with fulfilment as we move towards our goals.

In his early adulthood, Mandela set himself a seemingly impossible goal: to get rid of apartheid and establish South Africa as a democracy. It took him decades before he finally achieved that goal. But he was able to find fulfilment along the way, through continuously living by his values. With every step he took towards his goal, he knew he was standing for something – that he was doing something meaningful with his life – and that gave him fulfilment and satisfaction.

As Mandela writes in his autobiography, 'There are victories whose glory lies in the fact that they are only known to those who win them. This is particularly true of prison, where you must find consolation in being true to your ideals, even if no one else knows of it.'

VALUES AND THE 'P' WORD

One of the most common themes in this book is 'practice'. I've pointed out several times that we can't expect to *feel* confident in any activity until we have developed the necessary skills. And we can't develop those skills unless we practise. We also need to develop a capacity for mindfulness, so that we can engage fully in whatever we are doing, and defuse from unhelpful thought processes such as worrying, perfectionism and self-doubt. And obviously this also requires practice.

Unfortunately, it is much easier to talk about practice than to do it. Why? Because practice brings up uncomfortable thoughts and feelings. Even *thinking* about it often makes us uncomfortable. And human beings do not like feeling uncomfortable. So what do we tend to do? To avoid the discomfort, we don't do the practice. We either put it off until later, or we come up with reasons why we can't do it.

It's only natural that we do this. After all, in that moment when we decide to put it off or skip it, we usually get an instant feeling of relief: all those uncomfortable thoughts and feelings disappear. And that feels good, right? And everybody likes to feel good.

But here's the problem. Because we all like to have good feelings, we do what we can to avoid or get rid of unpleasant ones. And this all too easily becomes a habit. And then we start making unworkable choices: we do what gives us least discomfort in the short term, rather than what gives us most fulfilment in the long term.

Psychologists have a fancy term for this phenomenon. They call it 'experiential avoidance'. Experiential avoidance means trying hard to avoid or get rid of unwanted thoughts and feelings. Now, we are all experientially avoidant to some degree. I don't know anyone who loves having unpleasant thoughts and feelings, and never tries to avoid or get rid of them. But the more unwilling we are to make room for discomfort, the lower our quality of life. Indeed, high levels of experiential avoidance directly correlate with reduced performance, increased stress and higher risk of depression and anxiety.

Why should this be so? Because the more we try to avoid discomfort, the more we base our actions on how we *feel*, rather than on what is most important in life. In other words, we avoid doing things that are important and life-enhancing because we are unwilling to make room for the uncomfortable thoughts and feelings that show up. And the more we choose action that gives us short-term relief from discomfort, rather than doing what enriches our lives in the long term, the smaller and emptier our lives tend to become. We often call this 'living in the comfort zone'.

Here's a simple example of experiential avoidance: in reading this book, have you skipped any of the exercises? If so, why did you do that? Your mind might well have tried to justify this choice, by saying the exercise wasn't important, or you'd do it later – but isn't it the case that when you considered doing it, you felt some discomfort? And when you chose to skip it you felt some relief? If so, experiential avoidance has been dictating your choices.

And for most of us, this happens on a regular basis. When we put off or opt out of important goals and challenges, the chances are that we're not being true to ourselves; we're not behaving like the person we really want to be; we're not making choices in line with our long-term best interests.

So how do we get past this? How do we get ourselves to 'do the practice'? Do we read a Nike poster and then 'Just do it!'? Do we ask the universe to make it easy for us? Do we vividly imagine all our dreams coming true? Do we try to reprogramme our minds with positive thinking? These are all popular approaches, and you can be the judge of whether they work or not. What I can tell you is this: by the time they come to see me, most of my clients have tried these things and found they are not sustainable in the long term.

So what *is* sustainable? What can get us going and keep us going, even when we're tired, miserable, anxious, bored, frustrated, fearful or 'not in the mood'? What can motivate us to step out of our comfort zones into challenging situations that are guaranteed to bring up fear and anxiety? You guessed it: our values.

THE INNER COMPASS

As mentioned in chapter 1, our values are like a compass: they give us direction, guide our journey and help us stay on track. Our goals are things we want to accomplish along the way: to cross this river, climb that mountain, visit that castle or ski down that slope.

So suppose climbing Mount Everest is your goal. The values underlying it might be: courage, persistence, focus, doing your personal best, exercising and fitness, personal growth, connecting with nature, exploring and adventure. (Notice we could set a number of goals guided by these values; Everest is literally only one amongst millions.)

Now, obviously you can't climb Everest alone; you have to be part of a team. So there's another set of values to consider: what sort of teammate do you want to be? For example, do you want to be open-minded, flexible, considerate, friendly, helpful, respectful, reliable, loyal, honest, responsible and so on?

Notice that in both examples above, you can live by those values every step of the way towards your goals. And even if you never accomplish the goals of forming a team, or climbing Mount Everest, you can still live by those underlying values – courage, persistence, personal growth, open-mindedness, flexibility, responsibility and so on – and find plenty of fulfilment in doing so. (Of course, you'd feel disappointed if you didn't achieve your goals – but at least you'd have the satisfaction of knowing you'd been true to yourself, lived by your ideals, and behaved like the sort of person you want to be.)

In chapter 1, I asked you to consider how you would change if you developed genuine confidence: what goals you would set, what actions you would take, and how you would behave differently on an ongoing basis. In the next few chapters, we'll be revisiting these questions. Your answers are vitally important, because until now you've probably been stuck in the confidence gap: waiting until the day you *feel* confident before you start doing what really matters to you. And we've seen how that's a recipe for discontent: our lives get put on hold and we miss out on all sorts of opportunities. To win the game of confidence, we must play by the golden rule:

Rule 1: The actions *of confidence come first; the* feelings *of confidence come later.*

So here's where we're heading in the next few chapters. First, you'll clarify your values and goals and make sure that they're 'in sync'; that your goals are aligned with your values. Then you'll break those goals down into actions. Next you'll start taking those actions *mindfully*: engaging fully in what you do and unhooking yourself from unhelpful stories. As you do this, you will be *acting* with confidence: relying on yourself and trusting yourself to do what really matters. Finally, as you get better at what you do, and better at defusing from self-doubt and perfectionism, you are likely to notice the *feelings* of confidence appear.

Now, at some point in the process, you'll almost certainly get stuck. Feelings of fear and anxiety will arise, and you are highly likely to struggle with them. Fortunately, that's not a problem. Once you realize what has happened, you can use the mindfulness skill called 'expansion' to stop struggling with your feelings and handle them more effectively. That's what part 4 of this book is about. But given that we've only just started part 3, let's take . . .

A QUICK LOOK AT YOUR VALUES

There are many different ways to clarify our core values, and the exercise below was inspired by a similar one in the book *Curious* by Todd Kashdan. Below you'll find a list of common values, not all of which will be relevant to you. Keep in mind there is no such thing as a 'right' or 'wrong' value. It's a bit like our taste in pizzas. If you prefer ham and pineapple but I prefer salami and olives, that doesn't mean that my taste in pizzas is *right* and yours is *wrong*. It just means we have different tastes. And similarly, we may have different values. So read through the list below and write a letter next to each value: V = very important, Q = quite important, and N = not so important; and make sure to score *at least ten* of them as very important. (If you don't want to write in the book, you can download a pdf from the 'free resources' page on www. thehappinesstrap.co.uk.)

As you do this exercise, notice what your mind does. For example, if you score a value as very important, but you are currently behaving inconsistently with that value, your mind is likely to beat you up, or say, *Who are you kidding?*

COMMON VALUES

There is no such thing as a 'right' or 'wrong' value; this list is merely to get you thinking about what your own values

are. Mark each value as V, Q or N, where V= very important, Q = quite important, and N = not so important.

1. Acceptance: to be open to and accepting of myself, others, life and so on.

2. Adventure: to be adventurous; to actively seek, create or explore novel or stimulating experiences.

3. Assertiveness: to respectfully stand up for my rights and request what I want.

4. Authenticity: to be genuine and real; to be true to myself.

5. Beauty: to appreciate, create, nurture or cultivate beauty in myself, others, the environment and so on.

6. Caring: to be caring towards myself, others, the environment and so on.

7. Challenge: to keep challenging myself to grow, learn and improve.

8. Compassion: to act with kindness towards those who are suffering.

9. Contribution: to help or make a positive difference to myself or others.

10. Conformity: to be respectful and obedient of rules and obligations.

11. Connection: to engage fully in whatever I am doing, and be fully present with others.

12. Cooperation: to cooperate and collaborate with others.

13. Courage: to be brave; to persist in the face of fear, threat or difficulty.

14. Creativity: to be creative or innovative.

15. Curiosity: to be open-minded and interested; to explore and discover.

16. Encouragement: to reward behaviour that I value in myself or others.

17. Equality: to treat others as equal to myself, and vice versa.

18. Excitement: to seek, create and engage in activities that are exciting, stimulating or thrilling.

19. Fairness: to be fair to myself and others.

20. Fitness: to maintain or improve my fitness; to look after my physical and mental health and wellbeing.

21. Flexibility: to adjust and adapt readily to changing circumstances.

22. Freedom: to live freely; to choose how I live and behave, or help others do likewise.

23. Friendliness: to be friendly, companionable or agreeable towards others.

24. Forgiveness: to be forgiving towards myself and others.

25. Fun: to seek, create and engage in fun-filled activities.

26. Generosity: to be sharing and giving, to myself and others.

27. Gratitude: to be grateful for and appreciative of the positive aspects of myself, others and life.

28. Honesty: to be honest, truthful and sincere with myself and others.

29. Humour: to see and appreciate the humorous side of life.

30. Humility: to be humble or modest; to let my achievements speak for themselves.

31. Industry: to be industrious, hard-working, dedicated.

32. Independence: to support myself and choose my own way of doing things.

33. Intimacy: to open up, reveal and share myself – emotionally or physically – in my close personal elationships.
34. Justice: to uphold justice and fairness.
35. Kindness: to be kind, compassionate, considerate, nurturing or caring towards myself or others.
36. Love: to act lovingly or affectionately towards myself or others.
37. Mindfulness: to be conscious of, open to and curious about my here-and-now experience.
38. Order: to be orderly and organized.
39. Open-mindedness: to think things through, see things from others' points of view, and weigh evidence fairly.
40. Patience: to wait calmly and tolerantly for what I want.
41. Persistence: to continue resolutely, despite problems or difficulties.
42. Pleasure: to create and give pleasure to myself or others.
43. Power: to strongly influence or wield authority over others; to take charge, lead and organize.
44. Reciprocity: to build relationships in which there is a fair balance of giving and taking.
45. Respect: to be respectful towards myself and others; to be polite, considerate and show positive regard.
46. Responsibility: to be responsible and accountable for my actions.
47. Romance: to be romantic; to display and express love or strong affection.
48. Safety: to secure, protect, or ensure safety of myself or others.

49. Self-awareness: to be aware of my own thoughts, feelings and actions.
50. Self-care: to look after my health and wellbeing, and get my needs met.
51. Self-development: to keep growing, advancing or improving in knowledge, skills, character or life experience.
52. Self-control: to act in accordance with my own ideals.
53. Sensuality: to create, explore and enjoy experiences that stimulate the five senses.
54. Sexuality: to explore or express my sexuality.
55. Spirituality: to connect with things bigger than myself.
56. Skilfulness: to continually practise and improve my skills, and apply myself fully when using them.
57. Supportiveness: to be supportive, helpful, encouraging and available to myself or others.
58. Trust: to be trustworthy; to be loyal, faithful, sincere and reliable.
59. Insert your own unlisted value here.
60. Insert your own unlisted value here.

Once you've marked each value as V, Q, N (very, quite or not so important), go through all the Vs, and select out the top six that are most important to you. Mark each one with a 6, to show it's in your top six.

★★★

So what did that exercise reveal about the sort of person you want to be, the way you want to treat others and yourself, and what you want to stand for in life? (If you haven't done the exercise yet, what stopped you? Did you get hooked by 'Do it later' or 'Can't be bothered'? Or did an unpleasant feeling show up that you wanted to get rid of? Are you willing to go back and do it now, even though you may feel uncomfortable, and your mind's just given you some seemingly valid reasons not to do it?)

Very commonly, when we do this exercise, we discover significant gaps between our values and our actions. For example, Seb, the taxi driver who was avoiding sex with his wife, listed one of his top values as intimacy. Clearly there was a huge discrepancy between this core value and the way he was behaving towards his wife. The same was true for Claire, the shy receptionist who hadn't dated for years. One of her top values was authenticity, but she rarely allowed people to see the 'real' her, because she was afraid of rejection.

Similarly, in chapter 1 I introduced Alexis, a twenty-eight-year-old mother of two young boys, who said she would like to be more assertive with her domineering, hyper-critical mother-in-law. One of her core values was courage, and she did indeed act on this value in many areas of her life. For example, Alexis was a nurse, and before becoming a full-time mum, she had travelled the world widely and worked in field hospitals in war-torn parts of Africa. But when it came to standing up to her overbearing mother-in-law, she lost touch with her courage and shrank from the challenge.

When you find a gap between your values and your behaviour, there's no need to beat yourself up. This is simply a reminder that you are a normal human being, not a fictitious superhero. No one acts on their values all the time in every domain of life, and it's unrealistic to expect to do so. Sure, we can all get better at acting on our values, but we'll never be perfect. And keep in mind, the more destructive or self-defeating our behaviour, the more likely it is that we are acting inconsistently with our core values. For example, last night I had a huge argument with my wife. I lost my temper and said some really hurtful things to her. In that moment, my behaviour was both destructive and self-defeating; it was destructive to our relationship, and self-defeating in that it didn't help me to get the outcome I wanted. Was I acting on my core values during that argument? No way! I was acting totally inconsistently with three of my top six values: caring, connection and contribution. (Of course, once I calmed down, I reconnected with those values, promptly apologized and made up.)

Now I invite you to do another quick exercise: put this book down, grab a piece of paper, and write down those very important top six values. For the next few months, carry them around in your wallet or purse, and pull them out frequently to reflect on them. The more you are in touch with your core values, the more you can draw on them for inspiration and guidance.

AN IMPORTANT MESSAGE

Please be careful that you don't turn your values into rigid rules, such as: 'I have to be courageous at all times.' If your mind's using words like 'should', 'have to', 'must', 'ought', 'right' or 'wrong', then it's not reminding you of values, it's dictating the law. There's a huge difference between values and rules. For example, 'Thou shalt not kill' is *not* a value; it's a rigid rule. (A commandment, no less.) When we were children, the adults in our lives told us that if we follow this rule, we're 'good', and if we don't, we're 'bad'. But the values underlying this rigid rule are caring for and respecting human life. And there are many different ways to act on these values. (Please note, I am not suggesting for a moment that it's okay to break this rule. I am merely drawing the distinction between rules and values.)

Psychologist John Forsyth compares our values to a cube that constantly shifts position. No matter what the position, you can never see all faces of the cube simultaneously; some will be at the front, and others at the back. But the faces you can't see haven't ceased to exist; they're just not in the foreground. Similarly, in any given moment, some values are prominent, and others aren't. The values that we're *not* acting on haven't disappeared; it's just that in that moment, they're not a priority.

As we go through life, our rules about how to act on our values change dramatically, but the values themselves often don't change all that much. For example, ask a six-year-old boy how he would like to treat a little puppy dog, and he's likely to talk about feeding it, cuddling it and playing with it. What he's really talking about are the values of caring and nurturing. By the time that little boy becomes a thirty-six-year-old father of two children, he will have all sorts of sophisticated rules about how to look after his kids – bedtime routines, the best ways of encouraging them, rules about acceptable behaviour and so on – but the core values of caring and nurturing are the same.

The relative importance we place on our values usually changes enormously throughout our lives. For example, protecting your children is likely to be a top-priority value when they are young, vulnerable and defenceless. But by the time they are middle-aged with families of their own, this value, while it won't have disappeared, is likely to be somewhat less prominent. This means if you return to the exercise above in a year's time, you may find that some of the values you marked as not important have shifted to quite important or very important, and vice versa; and your top six list may have altered dramatically. (On the other hand, it may not change much at all; everyone's experience is unique.)

A word of warning: watch out for perfectionist hooks such as 'I *have to* live by my values at all times.' You don't *have to* do any such thing. Values are simply words that express the way you ideally want to behave. You don't *have to* act on them; it's a personal choice. In ACT we encourage you to use your values as a guide, because this generally leads to fulfilment and vitality; but we wouldn't want you to turn them into a set of rigid rules for controlling your life. Steve Hayes, the creator of ACT, has a good way of saying this, which gives us the fifth rule of the confidence game:

Rule 5: Hold your values lightly, but pursue them vigorously.

If we follow this rule flexibly and mindfully (as opposed to rigidly and automatically), it will allow us to escape from . . .

chapter 12

the success trap

What does the word 'success' mean to you?

When you hear 'She is very successful' or 'He's made a success of himself', what does that conjure up for you? Our society generally defines success in terms of achieving goals: fame, wealth, status and respect; a big house, a luxury car, a prestigious job, a huge salary. When people achieve these things, our society tends to label them as 'successful'. But if we buy into this popular notion of success, we set ourselves up for a lot of unnecessary suffering.

How so? Well, this view of success inevitably pulls us into the 'goal-focused life', where we are always striving to achieve the next goal. We may strive for more money, a larger house, a better neighbourhood, smarter clothes, a slimmer body, bigger muscles, more status, more fame, more respect and so on. We may strive to win this game or tournament, or make that sale, or get that promotion, or win that contract, or find a more attractive partner, or buy that smart car, or get that qualification, or earn that university degree.

And the illusion is, 'When I achieve this goal, then I will be successful.'

There are at least three big problems associated with going through life this way. First, there's no guarantee you will achieve those goals, or they may be a long way off – which leads to chronic frustration and disappointment. Second, even if you do achieve them, they will not give you lasting happiness; usually they give you a brief moment of pleasure, satisfaction or joy – and then you start to focus on the next goal. Third, if you buy into this notion of success, it will put you under tremendous pressure – because you have to keep on achieving and achieving to maintain it. As long as you can keep achieving those goals, then you are 'successful' – 'a winner', 'a high achiever', 'a champion'. But if you stop achieving, then you are no longer successful; you are a 'has-been', 'a failure' or 'a loser'.

It is this popular notion of success that creates the commonplace problem of 'fragile self-esteem'. Fragile self-esteem is very common in high-performing professionals. These high achievers often develop a strong positive self-image based on their performance: as long as they perform well, they have high self-esteem. But as soon as their performance drops, their self-esteem comes tumbling down: from 'winner' to 'loser', from 'high achiever' to 'failure'.

If we live our lives ruled by this definition of success, we are doomed to stress and misery (punctuated by brief moments of joy when we achieve a goal). So I invite you to consider a radically different definition: *True success is living by your values.*

This definition makes our lives ever so much easier. Why? Because in any moment, we can act on our values – yes, even if we've neglected them for years. *Hey presto*: instant success!

This concept is especially useful if your goals are a long way off: you don't have to wait until you've achieved them; you can be successful right now through living by your values. Suppose you want to change career and become a cardiac surgeon. You're looking at a minimum of ten years before you can achieve this goal. That's a long time. But suppose the core value underlying that goal is 'helping others'; you can successfully act on that value over and over, all day, every day, for the rest of your life – even if you never become a cardiac surgeon.

Consider this quote from Martin Luther King, Jr: 'I have a dream that my four little children will one day live in a nation where they will not be judged by the colour of their skin, but by the content of their character.' This comes from his famous speech, delivered on the steps of the Lincoln Memorial, Washington DC, to a crowd of 200,000 civil rights protesters, on 28 August 1963. By the popular notion of 'success equals achieving your goals', Martin Luther King was *not* successful. He did not achieve his goal of equal rights for people of all skin colours. And yet we remember, admire and respect him. Why? Because he stood for something: he lived by his values!

When living by our values becomes the definition of success, it means we can be successful right now. All we need to do is act on our values. From this perspective, the mother who gives up her career to act on her values around nurturing and supporting her children is far more successful than the CEO who earns millions but completely neglects his values around being there for his kids. Albert Einstein put it this way: 'Try not to become a man of success, but rather try to become a man of value.' And Helen Keller put it like this: 'I long to accomplish a great and noble task, but it is my chief duty to accomplish small tasks as if they were great and noble.' So next time your mind is beating you up for not being successful enough, try saying 'Thanks mind!' And then ask yourself 'What's a tiny little thing I can do right now that's consistent with my values?' Then do it: instant success!

JOURNEY AND DESTINATION

We can now list another 'right rule' for the confidence game:

Rule 6: True success is living by your values.

Playing by this rule doesn't mean we give up on our goals. It means we use our values to set our goals, and to sustain us as we move towards them. I often hear people say, 'It's the journey that counts, not the destination', but I don't agree. The destination *is* important: a journey from New York to Paris is not the same as a journey from New York to Shanghai. The point is this: all you have in any moment is the journey itself, because the instant you actually reach your destination, it is, by definition, no longer your destination. The moment you reach Paris, you're in Paris. And then a split second later, you're on a new journey, with a new destination: the hotel you're staying at. So why not appreciate every moment of the journey, rather than focusing solely on the destination?

You may be more familiar with this concept in terms of 'process' and 'outcome'. 'Process' is the way you go about doing something. 'Outcomes' are the results of what you've done. If you want to develop genuine confidence, perform at your peak, and find maximal fulfilment in what you do, you need to commit to the process, engaging in it fully and detaching from the outcome.

Again, that doesn't mean giving up on the goal; it simply means shifting the emphasis: instead of obsessing about the outcome, you get passionate about the process; about getting the most out of it, and doing it to the best of your ability.

One of my clients, Ginny, was learning to paint, but she didn't enjoy it very much because she spent the whole time fretting about what the finished painting would look like – obsessing about the outcome. So I asked her what she could get out of the process, even if the finished result wasn't what she wanted. Ginny identified that she could learn how to use colour, tone, light and composition, and how to create different textures with the paintbrush. Next I asked her what values she wanted to act on in every moment of painting. She identified learning and being creative. Finally I asked her to go back to her painting and get passionate about the process: to embrace it as an opportunity for learning new skills and being creative. Ginny soon found that the more she engaged in the process and detached from the outcome, the more rewarding the experience was. Soon she was able to enjoy the painting without getting hung up on the end result. And paradoxically, her paintings turned out much better!

So here's another rule for the confidence game:

Rule 7: Don't obsess on the outcome; get passionate about the process.

A TALE OF TWO MOUNTAIN CLIMBERS

Hank and Jake are both passionate mountain climbers, both equally skilled. But they have very different attitudes to climbing.

Hank is totally goal-focused. All that matters to him is reaching the top of the mountain in the shortest possible time. Every step of the way, all he cares about is reaching the summit. He is so intent on getting to the top, he can hardly bear to stop and take a rest. And when he does force himself to take a break, all he can think about is that ticking clock, and how much further there is still to go. As he climbs, there is little joy or satisfaction in the process; he is constantly pressuring himself to get to the top, all too aware that he's still not there.

When he finally reaches the summit, he is delighted. He has done it. Woohoo! A moment of crowning glory. For one brief instant, while he takes in the view, the pressure is off. But it doesn't last long. The moment he sets off back down, once again his goal dominates all else: all that matters is to get there as fast as possible.

In stark contrast, Jake's approach to climbing the mountain is values-focused. He has the same goal as Hank: to reach the peak in a good time. However, he is much more in touch with the values underlying his goal: developing his skills, appreciating nature, acting courageously, challenging himself, exercising his body, exploring and adventuring. As he climbs, he savours every moment of the ascent. He is not constantly thinking about the summit and pressuring himself to get there; he is living in the present moment, totally engaged in what he is doing. Regardless of where he is on the mountain – bottom, middle or top – he is mindfully acting on his values. When he stops for a rest, he takes in the view and appreciates how far he has come. When he reaches the top, he is exhilarated; the view is breathtaking. And whether he is going upwards or back down, he savours every bit of the journey.

Now suppose the weather turns nasty, and they can't make it to the top of the mountain; they have to turn back. Both climbers are disappointed; they failed to achieve their goal. But Jake handles it much better than Hank. Why? Because Jake has found the climb fulfilling in itself; he got to develop and apply his skills, to explore and be adventurous, to challenge himself and to appreciate nature. So even though it didn't turn out the way he wished, Jake regards it as a successful and rewarding outing. Hank, in contrast, is eaten up with disappointment and regards the outing as a failure. Why? Because he didn't achieve his goal. All he can think about is when he can come back and try again.

This is the difference between the values-focused life and the goal-focused life. Jake gets to achieve his goals and appreciate every step along the way. And even if he doesn't achieve his goals, he still gets huge satisfaction from living by his values.

By contrast, Hank lives in a state of self-imposed pressure and chronic frustration. It's all about the goals – and there's no satisfaction unless he achieves them. And even if he does achieve those goals, he experiences only a brief moment of joy and then it's back to the pressure and frustration. For sure, some people do manage to achieve a lot with this extreme focus on goals – but the costs are usually huge in terms of stress, dissatisfaction and ultimately psychological 'burnout' or physical ill-health.

Values are wonderful things. They don't just provide a means for instant success; they also behave like a sort of . . .

chapter 13

magic glue

Does the name *Tiktaalik* mean anything to you?

No, it's not a character from *The Lord of the Rings*. *Tiktaalik* is a very old fish. Three hundred and seventy-five million years old, to be precise. The name means 'large freshwater fish' in the language of the Inuit people, who inhabit the Nunavut territory of the Arctic. Which is precisely where Neil Shubin and his colleagues discovered their ancient fossil. And when they announced their discovery, in April 2006, it made world headlines.

You see, *Tiktaalik* has a flat head with very sharp teeth, rather like the head of a crocodile. It also has scales and fins, rather like a fish. And yet it is neither a reptile nor a fish. Shubin had discovered a so-called 'missing link': a creature that represented an intermediate evolutionary stage between fish and reptiles.

Now whether or not you believe in evolution or give a damn about fossil-hunting, you have to admire Shubin's persistence. He and his team had to make no fewer than four Arctic expeditions over six years to find this fossil, spending day after day, week after week searching through frozen soil in the desolate vastness of Ellesmere Island: a task arguably harder than searching for the proverbial needle in the haystack.

I read about Shubin's adventures in his fascinating book, *Your Inner Fish*, and was particularly intrigued by his early experiences in fossil-hunting. His first expedition, as a total novice, was in the Arizona desert. They were looking for tiny fossils, each no more than a few centimetres in length. Each day, Shubin would set off enthusiastically into the desert, and eagerly inspect every rock he found for scraps of bone. And each day he would come back empty-handed, while the other palaeontologists returned with bags full of bones.

This went on for several weeks. Then Shubin had a bright idea: instead of going solo, he would tag along with the team leader, Chuck Schaff. So each day thereafter, as they trawled the desert together, Shubin would pick Schaff's brain for useful tips. Unfortunately, while Schaff was incredibly cooperative, and provided a veritable goldmine of information, it didn't seem to be of any help.

Shubin found it all very embarrassing. He and Schaff would look at the same patch of desert floor, and Shubin would see nothing but rocks and sand, whereas Schaff would spot a wealth of tiny teeth, jaws, bones and bits of skull.

Schaff's recurring advice was to 'look for something different'; something that had a different texture to rock, a different surface, a different form, a different way of glistening under the sun.

Well, Shubin looked and looked for 'something different' – but he didn't find it. His embarrassment grew ever stronger, as day after day he came home with nothing, while Schaff returned with bags of fossils.

Then one day, after many weeks of this, Shubin finally saw his first piece of tooth, glinting in the sunlight. Resting on a pile of sandstone rubble, he could see it, clear as daylight. He had finally trained his eyes to do what he wanted; now he could see the difference between rock and bone. He writes: 'All of a sudden, the desert floor exploded with bone.' Where previously he could see nothing but rock, there were now tiny fossil fragments all over the place. It was as if he had donned 'a special new pair of glasses and a spotlight was shining on all the different pieces of bone'. From this day on, Shubin always came back loaded with fossils.

THE MAGIC GLUE

Our values are like magic glue. They glue together the tiniest little actions to the biggest, long-term goals. Shubin's values included exploring, curiosity, adventure, persistence, endurance, commitment, learning new skills and challenging himself. Those values glued together every second of every day of every week, searching in vain for fossils in the desert. Day after day, he failed to achieve his goal – but he lived by his values, and despite his embarrassment and disappointment, he had the satisfaction of doing something personally meaningful. And then, one day, he *did* achieve his goal. And even though it was just a tiny fragment of tooth, to Shubin 'it was as glorious as the biggest dinosaur in the halls of any museum'.

But it would never have happened without committed action. Only through serving his time scouring the desert could he develop those 'fossil-hunter eyes'. And the same values sustained him all the way from that first fragment of tooth in the Arizona desert to the discovery of *Tiktaalik* many years later.

So let's now look at your life and see if we can mix up a batch of magic glue. For the exercises that follow, we're going to divide your life into four domains: Love, Work, Play and Health. The Love segment refers to all the time and effort you invest in your deepest relationships: with your children, parents, partner, and close friends and relatives. The Play segment refers to all the time and effort you invest in rest and relaxation, hobbies, creativity, sport and all forms of leisure, recreation and entertainment. The Work segment refers to all the time and effort you invest in paid work, unpaid work (such as volunteering or domestic duties), and studying, education and apprenticeships. The Health segment refers to all the time and effort you invest in looking after your physical, psychological, emotional or spiritual health and wellbeing.

These are arbitrary divisions and I leave it to you to decide exactly what goes where. For example, if you're doing a course for fun rather than to enhance your career, you'd consider that 'play', rather than 'work'. If you earn your main income from playing football, you'd class that as 'work' rather than 'play'. Now, in order to find the glue in these domains, we'll need to do a spot of mind-reading.

THE MIND-READING MACHINE
I want you to imagine that I have invented an amazing device that enables you to read the mind of anybody on the planet. I hook you up to the machine and turn the dial. Suddenly a picture appears on the screen. It's an image of someone who is very important to you in the life domain of love. Just pause for a moment, and conjure up an image of this person.

***

Now I pull a lever, and suddenly you are reading this person's mind. And they just happen to be thinking about *you*. They are thinking about your character: about what sort of personal strengths and qualities you have, and what you mean to them, and the role that you have played in their life. They are *not* thinking about all the goals you have achieved; they are thinking about the sort of person you are, and what you stand for in life. And I'd like you now to imagine, if dreams could come true, then what would you love to hear this person thinking?

Note: this is an exercise in imagination; a fantasy to help you uncover your values. You are not trying to realistically predict what this person would truly be thinking; you are fantasizing about what you'd love them to be thinking if magic could happen. So please close your eyes or fix on a spot, and take a couple of minutes to imagine this scenario. What would you love them to be thinking about you?

★★★

Please write down a few words about what you imagined.

★★★

Now choose someone else who is important to you in the life domain of work. And imagine a similar scenario to that above. They pop up on the screen, and you tune in to their thoughts. They are thinking about what sort of character you have, what you mean to them, and the role you have played in their life. Once again, close your eyes and for a couple of minutes just fantasize. Imagine: if dreams could come true, what would you love to hear this person thinking about you?

★★★

Now write a few words about what you imagined.

★★★

Choose a third person who is important to you in the life domain of play, and run through the exercise again. As you tune in to their thoughts about what sort of character you have, what you mean to them, and the role you have played in their life, what would you love to hear them thinking?

★★★

Now write a few words about what you imagined.

★★★

For this last part, there is a special attachment on the machine that allows you to hear what your own body is thinking. (Yes, I know that sounds crazy, but this is an imaginative exercise so anything can happen.) Your body pops on to the screen and you hear its thoughts about how you treat it, what you do for it, and how you look after it. If dreams could come true, what would you love to hear your body thinking?

★★★

Now write a few words about what you imagined.

TUNING IN TO YOUR HEART

There are no right answers to the exercise above. It is there to help you discover what really matters to you, about the sort of person you want to be. (And if you didn't do it, notice how you're making a choice to avoid short-term discomfort rather than doing what will help you find long-term fulfilment. Don't beat yourself up about it; we all do this at times. Just notice it and learn from it; we often fail to realize just how much of our lives are organized around avoiding discomfort. And just consider: are you willing to go back and do it? It only takes eight minutes in total (four times two minutes).

When Cleo, the shy scientist, completed this exercise, she found the same values cropping up again and again: she wanted to be warm, open, genuine, supportive and authentic. However, in social situations she would all too often clam up and reveal little of her true thoughts and feelings, so she rarely came across as the warm, open, genuine person she wanted to be. Another important value for Cleo was courage. She realized that each time she avoided a social event, she was acting inconsistently with this value. Clarifying these core values was an important step for Cleo. It not only laid the foundation for setting goals – as you'll see shortly – it also provided ongoing inspiration for the journey ahead.

I invite you now to draw on what you've just discovered, as well as the top six values list from chapter 11, to complete the form below. I call it The Values Window, because it gives you a lookout into the life you want. (And as usual, if you're totally unwilling to write your answers down, then please at least think about them; and if you don't want to write in the book, you can copy the form out, or download a copy from the 'free resources' page at www. thehappinesstrap.co.uk.)

In the Values Window, there are four frames corresponding to the major life domains of love, work, play and health. In each frame, please clarify your values, then your goals. Short-term goals are things you'd like to achieve in the next few days and weeks. Medium-term goals are things you'd like to achieve in the next few weeks and months. Long-term goals are things you'd like to achieve over months and years.

Make sure your goals are specific, rather than vague and fuzzy. Here's an example of a specific goal: 'On Thursday night I will sit at my computer from 8 p.m. to 11 p.m. and draw up the first draft of a business plan.' Here's an example of a vague and fuzzy

The Values Window

LOVE (Deepest, most meaningful relationships – including children, partner, parents, close friends and relatives) My Values: Short-Term Goals: Medium-Term Goals: Long-Term Goals:	**WORK** (Paid work, studying/education, apprenticeships, and unpaid work such as volunteering, or domestic duties) My Values: Short-Term Goals Medium-Term Goals Long-Term Goals
PLAY (Rest and relaxation, hobbies, creativity, sport, and all forms of leisure, recreation and entertainment) My Values: Short-Term Goals: Medium-Term Goals: Long-Term Goals:	**HEALTH** (Physical, psychological, emotional or spiritual health and wellbeing) My Values: Short-Term Goals Medium-Term Goals Long-Term Goals

goal: 'I'll think some more about my business ideas.' Here is another example, just to be clear. Specific: 'On Sunday night after dinner, I will spend an hour practising my talk for the Monday morning meeting.' Vague: 'In future, I'll practise my talks a bit more.' This is an important distinction; a wealth of research shows that we are far more likely to achieve a specific, well-defined goal than a vague and fuzzy one.

So using your values as a guide, please now set some specific and meaningful goals. And as you do this exercise, please notice what your mind has to say, and the feelings that arise inside your body.

YOU CAN'T DO IT ALL AT ONCE!

Have you completed The Values Window, either mentally or on paper? If so, pause for ten seconds, and notice what your mind is saying.

***

Is it jumping for joy, or telling you it's all too hard? If your mind's anything like mine, it's doing the latter. When we start setting goals, our minds can easily get overwhelmed: 'I can't possibly do all these things; it's too much. Aaaaaargggghhhh!' So if that's what your mind is doing, please thank it and carry on reading.

If you want to carve a sculpture from a block of marble, you can't chip away at every part of the block simultaneously. You have to choose somewhere to start. You chip away at that area for a while, and then once you have made some progress, you move on to another part. The same holds true for shaping our lives. If we try working away at every part of them simultaneously, we'll get over-whelmed, and we'll either give up or make a hash of it.

So I invite you now to read through what you've written, and select just one domain of life – love, work, play or health – and no more than two or three short-term goals. Once you've made some progress with these goals, then you can choose some others to work on – either from the same life domain, or a different one. And you can keep on doing this for the rest of your life. Naturally, at times you'll focus more on one domain than others, but hopefully over time you'll take care of them all.

After filling in the values window, Cleo chose to focus first and foremost on the domain of love. Here's how it looked on her worksheet:

LOVE
My values: To be warm, open, genuine, supportive and authentic in my social interactions. To be more courageous, and to act on what's in my heart rather than being ruled by my fear.

Short-term goals: Monday morning, ask two co-workers that I hardly ever talk to about what they did on the weekend, and I'll tell them what I did.

Medium-term goals: Join a book club. Contribute more in conversations, and reveal more of my own opinions and ideas. Practise asking open-ended questions. Practise telling anecdotes.

Long-term goals: To build an active social life, going out at least once a week. To make at least two or three new friends within the next year.

On your own worksheet, if you've written a lot more than in the above example, that's not a problem; but if you've written a lot less, that probably indicates you need to invest a bit more time and effort. Once you've completed the exercise, contemplate your goals and notice the thoughts and feelings that show up. Do you feel any sense of fear, anxiety, trepidation or nervousness? If so, good; you'll be needing it for the next part of the book.

part four

taming your fear

chapter 14

the fear trap

At the age of nineteen, Albert Ellis was terrified of rejection by women.

Of course, at that point in his life, Ellis had no idea that he would one day become one of the most influential psychologists of the twentieth century. It didn't even figure in his wildest dreams. What he *did* dream about was getting over his fear. So what did he do about it?

For one month, Ellis visited the New York Botanical Gardens every day and forced himself to talk to every attractive woman he encountered. Fearful though he was, somehow he managed to open his mouth and get the words out. And by the end of the month, he had asked over a hundred women for a date. And not one single one of them said 'yes'!

But Ellis did not see this as a failure. On the contrary, he regarded it as a great success. Why? Because by this point, he had completely overcome his fear of rejection. He had learned that fear was nothing more nor less than an unpleasant feeling; that it couldn't stop him from doing what he wanted. It was a profound insight which freed him to live a lifetime of adventure. (I debated whether to include this example in the book, because many women dislike being hassled in this way, and this could make Ellis sound a bit like a pick-up artist – but I chose to include it anyway. I am not advocating or condoning this behaviour, merely using it as a dramatic example of someone overcoming a deeply held fear.)

A DANGEROUS BEAST?

Imagine you've grown up in a weird community, and you've been taught that sheep are the most dangerous animals on the planet: that they have huge, razor-sharp teeth which can tear you to shreds; that they love nothing more than to kill and eat humans; and they can leap higher than a three-storey house.

Suppose you completely believe this. And one day, you are out walking through the countryside when you suddenly catch sight of a sheep. It's staring at you from behind a small wooden fence. How would you feel? Nervous? Anxious? Terrified?

This may seem like a far-fetched fantasy, but it's rather like the way we've all been raised to think about fear. From a young age we've been educated to believe that fear is 'bad': that it's a sign of weakness, that it's unnatural, that successful people don't have it, that it holds us back in life, and that we need to reduce it or get rid of it. And we all too readily believe this stuff, because a) the brainwashing starts when we're naive little kids, and b) fear feels so unpleasant, it seems to make sense that it would be bad for us.

So as a result, we have learned to fear our own fear. We have become anxious about our anxiety. We're nervous about our nervousness. Spot the vicious cycle, anyone?

WHAT IS FEAR?

Consult a few dictionaries or textbooks and you'll usually find fear defined something like this: 'A feeling of agitation or apprehension, in response to a real or imagined threat.' Throughout this book, I've been using the word 'fear' very loosely, as a catch-all phrase which covers all its relatives: anxiety, 'nerves', panic, stress, self-doubt, insecurity and so on. In this section of the book, we are going to focus on the *physical* aspects of fear; the sensations and feelings in our bodies: sweaty hands, racing heart, jelly legs, butterflies in the stomach, lump in the throat, dry mouth, tense neck, fidgety feet and so on.

Obviously, thoughts play an important role in creating, maintaining and exacerbating our fears, and the best way to deal with those is through defusion. In other words, when your mind conjures up a scary thought, image or memory, notice it, name it, and neutralize it. However, in ACT we use a different mindfulness skill to deal with feelings and sensations in our bodies. It's called 'expansion', and I'm going to cover it in detail in the next two chapters. But first, let's consider how we typically react to fear.

AUTOPILOT AND AVOIDANCE

Most of us aren't too good at handling painful emotions such as anger, fear, sadness and guilt. We typically have two modes of responding to them: autopilot mode and avoidance mode.

Autopilot mode

In autopilot mode, we are at the mercy of our emotions. It's as if we are robots and the emotions control our every move. Anger shows up and suddenly we are lashing out, yelling abuse or stomping our feet. Fear shows up and we run, withdraw or hide from our challenges. When you're on automatic pilot, you are not mindful of where you are and what you are doing, and you are definitely not in touch with your values. Instead, your emotions are running the show; jerking you around as if you were a puppet on a string. Unfortunately this creates the illusion that strong emotions are dangerous, which then feeds the myth that we can't act the way we want unless we can control the way we feel.

Avoidance mode

You don't have to be a top psychologist to figure out that humans like feeling good. None of us enjoy unpleasant feelings. And let's face it, under most circumstances, fear is an unpleasant feeling. (I say 'most circumstances' because at times we may hand over good money in order to have this very feeling: for example, if we watch a scary movie, read a thriller, or take a ride on a roller-coaster.) Given that fear usually feels unpleasant, and our society also teaches us that it's 'bad', it's only natural we try to avoid or get rid of it. You may recall that this is known as 'experiential avoidance'.

In avoidance mode, we do whatever we can to get rid of or avoid unpleasant feelings. Common tactics we use include distraction, opting out, thinking strategies and substance use. Let's quickly look at each of these methods.

Distraction

We try hard to distract ourselves from our feelings through books, movies, computer games, TV, socializing, music, sport, exercise, crossword puzzles, cooking, cleaning, sex, gambling, sleeping, throwing ourselves into work, focusing on other people's problems and so on.

Opting out

Challenging situations give rise to uncomfortable feelings. So in order to avoid those feelings, we opt out of challenging situations.

We quit, withdraw, procrastinate, escape, or stay away from people, places, events, situations and activities that we find challenging.

Thinking strategies

When we have unpleasant feelings, we often try to think our way out of them. Here are a few of the more common thinking strategies we use: blaming others, analysing why we feel this way, thinking about something more pleasant, denying that we're in pain, positive thinking, optimistic thinking, positive affirmations, challenging negative thoughts, fantasizing about the future, planning revenge, planning to escape, beating ourselves up, telling ourselves we 'shouldn't be feeling this way', telling ourselves to 'snap out of it', active problem-solving, telling ourselves 'It's not fair', wondering 'Why me?', imagining 'If only', rehashing the past and so on.

Substance use

We all at times put substances into our bodies in an attempt to get rid of unpleasant feelings and replace them with more pleasant ones. Which of the following do you use: painkillers like aspirin and paracetamol, drinks such as tea or coffee, herbal or naturopathic remedies, prescription medications, alcohol, tobacco, marijuana or other illicit drugs, chocolate, pizza, ice cream, hamburgers or chips?

So what's the problem?

At times, we all operate in avoidance or autopilot mode. And this isn't always a problem. But the more habitual it becomes and the more time we spend in these modes, the more problems they create.

For example, the more I go through my day on autopilot, the less control I have. When fear and anxiety show up, they dictate my choices. I don't stop to consciously reflect on my options; I do whatever the fear tells me to do. If Albert Ellis had been operating on autopilot, he never would have spoken to those women. He would have let fear dictate his actions, and steered clear of such challenging situations.

What about avoidance mode? Well, any of those common methods for avoiding painful feelings – distraction, opting out, thinking strategies and substance use – can readily create problems. If we use them sparingly and wisely, these methods are fine. But if we use them excessively and rigidly, there will be many undesirable consequences.

First let's consider *distraction*. The more I invest my time and energy in doing things to distract myself from my feelings, the less time and energy I have to invest in the things that make life rich, full and meaningful. Not to mention that some distractions, such as gambling or shopping, have big financial costs; and others, such as partying hard or working hard, can have big health costs over time.

What about *opting out*? The more I use this as a strategy for avoiding fear, the smaller my life gets. I avoid taking risks. I avoid stepping out of my comfort zone. I avoid facing my challenges. I get stuck in a rut and miss out on all sorts of opportunities.

One form of opting out is procrastination: putting it off until later. While this is fine at times, if I do it too much, important issues do not get dealt with, problems do not get resolved, and my to-do list grows bigger and bigger (which generates extra anxiety).

When we over-rely on *thinking strategies,* there are many costs. A particularly big one is that we spend a lot of time in our heads instead of engaging in our lives. Others depend on the strategy used. Blaming others leads to relationship conflicts. Fantasizing about the future leads to discontent with the present. Beating ourselves up just makes us miserable. Positive thinking and challenging thoughts lead to frustration and disappointment when they don't have the desired effects.

And if we over-rely on *substance use*, the costs to our physical health vary from addiction to lung cancer to obesity.

But arguably the biggest cost of all is that the more we avoid our own fear, the bigger it grows and the more influence it has over our actions. We get stuck in the fear trap: the greater our efforts to get rid of fear, the greater our fear becomes, and the more negatively it affects our lives. For example, Seb tried to avoid his fear of sexual failure by refusing to have sex with his wife. In the short term, this strategy helped him avoid his fear, but in the long term, his fear of failure just grew bigger – and he therefore became even more reluctant to have sex. By the time he sought help, he'd avoided making love to his wife for four years, and it had turned into a major source of conflict within their relationship.

THE FEAR TRAP

Have you ever heard the saying, 'Get back on the horse'? Personally, I've never fallen from a horse, but I've been told it is pretty scary. Immediately after a big fall, most people would have some fear of getting back on – especially if they were injured when they fell. But the sooner you get back on and start riding again, the sooner you will regain your confidence. What happens if you don't remount the horse; if you put it off, week after week, saying, 'I'll start again, next week'? The longer you put off riding, the greater your fear grows.

If you want to get back into horse-riding, then you have to face your fear; you have to 'get back on the horse'. Psychologists refer to this concept as 'exposure' (and it has nothing to do with taking your clothes off in public). 'Exposure' basically means staying in contact with whatever you're afraid of until you get used to it. And it has more positive impact on behaviour than any other tool, technique, or strategy known to humankind.

You've probably seen documentaries where people overcome their phobias. Let's say the subject is terrified of spiders: he panics whenever he sees one, and he won't go anywhere near them. He lives his life doing whatever he can to avoid spiders. He avoids looking at pictures of them. He closes his eyes if they appear in movies. He even tries to avoid talking about them. The problem is, the more he avoids anything to do with spiders, the more afraid he becomes of them.

To get him over his fear, a psychologist 'exposes' him to spiders in a gentle step-by-step programme. First he looks at pictures of spiders. Then he watches videos of spiders. Then he looks at realistic toy spiders. Then he looks at dead spiders in display cases. Then he looks at living spiders crawling around inside glass jars. Eventually he can even hold a living spider in his hand. (Of course, most people wouldn't go quite that far, unless they planned to get into spider-breeding or something.) This step-by-step approach is known as 'graded exposure'. And you can see that it is the very opposite of avoidance.

But suppose what we fear is not something outside us, like a horse, a spider or a mad axeman. Suppose what we fear is an emotion, feeling or sensation. As long as we go through life trying hard to avoid that feeling, we will never overcome our fear of it.

You may recall the term 'experiential avoidance': the ongoing effort to avoid or get rid of unwanted thoughts and feelings. Experiential avoidance is like an emotional amplifier: it takes our fear and makes it bigger and bigger. And this then leads us to try even harder to avoid it. Which makes it even bigger, and so on and so on. Thus the more experientially avoidant we are, the more firmly stuck we are in the fear trap.

So what is the alternative? Should we just grit our teeth, put up with the fear and force ourselves to go through with it? Well, we could do that, but I wouldn't recommend it. There is another way of responding to fear that is radically different from almost everything our society encourages us to do. We don't 'put up with it' or 'tolerate it'. We don't suppress it or deny its existence. We don't distract ourselves from it. We don't try to talk ourselves out of it. We don't try to reduce it or eliminate it with self-hypnosis or other techniques. We don't try to make it go away with medication, herbal remedies or food or alcohol. We don't try to pretend it's not there (the so-called 'fake it till you make it' approach).

So what do we do? All we need do is give it . . .

chapter 15

plenty of space

A bleak desert wasteland populated by lost souls. Here there is no escape from the ravages of the scorching sun, the plagues of flies, and the ever-present threat of violence. Murder and mayhem, rape and revenge, torture and torment: these are not freak occurrences, but parts of the daily routine for those who live here.

If you've seen *The Proposition*, you'll know what I'm talking about. It is a grim and extremely violent Western (brilliant, but horrific) set in the Australian outback in 1880. It was filmed on location in the middle of summer, and the actors had to cope with blistering heat and huge swarms of flies constantly buzzing all around them.

Now, obviously the actors couldn't keep waving the flies away, or they'd ruin all the shots; they had to let the flies crawl on their faces without reacting. This also made it more authentic; the historical advisers on the film believed that people in that era would have been so used to flies crawling all over them, they wouldn't have been constantly shooing them away. One of the lead actors in the film, Ray Winstone, said he'd always wondered how those lions in wildlife documentaries seemed so oblivious to all the flies. However, after a few days of filming, he got used to them. Soon he was able to let the flies be there without being bothered by them. He said they felt 'like feathers stroking my face'.

That's a pretty amazing attitude shift, isn't it? Under normal circumstances, we try as hard as we can to get rid of flies. We swipe at them, swat them and spray them. We may install clever flytraps, put up flyscreens, and do whatever we can to keep them out of our houses. And this is only natural; we know they are dirty and carry germs, and if they contaminate our food we can get sick. So of course we hate the idea of letting them crawl on us. And yet, when Ray Winstone defused from all those thoughts and mindfully noticed the actual sensations of flies crawling on him, he discovered it was nowhere near as bad as he'd expected.

Now don't worry, I'm not going to ask you to let flies crawl on you. But I'd like you to consider this possibility: suppose you could change your attitude towards your own fear in the same way Ray Winstone did with the flies. Suppose you could defuse from all those thoughts about how bad or unpleasant your fear is, and how much you dislike it – and instead of trying to make it go away, you non-judgementally noticed the physical sensations.

If your mind is saying something like, 'Why would I bother?', the answer is very simple. Trying to get rid of your fear takes up a lot of energy and is very distracting (like constantly trying to shoo away flies); it's hard to engage fully in your life while you're busy struggling with your feelings.

MYTH-BUSTING TIME AGAIN!

At this point, many of my clients start to protest, especially if they've been struggling with performance anxiety. They trot out the myth that high levels of anxiety impair performance – and therefore it needs to be reduced. Unfortunately, this deeply held belief is not only regurgitated in many books on business and sports psychology, but also in many popular self-help books. Luckily, there's plenty of published research to show it's not true.

For example, common sense suggests that if you feel less anxious during academic tests, then you'll perform better. But in 1988, psychologists A. R. Rich and D. K. Woolever published some fascinating research that clearly showed this is *not* the case. They showed that when sitting academic tests, most people have similar levels of anxiety. And what determines their performance is not their anxiety level, but their capacity for task-focused attention. In other words, if they could engage fully in the exam, instead of getting distracted by their own thoughts and feelings, they performed well *no matter how anxious they were.*

Other published studies in the fields of both athletic and sexual performance show similar results. (You can find these studies, by the psychologists D. H. Barlow, T. J. Bruce, S. Hanton, L. Hardy, G. Jones and A. B. J. Swain, listed in the references section at the back of the book.) Performance is not related to levels of anxiety, but to capacity for task-focused attention. Athletes and lovers who engage fully in the task perform best. Those who get distracted by their own thoughts and feelings perform worst.

So when you put all your mindfulness skills together – when you unhook from unhelpful thoughts, make room for unpleasant feelings and engage fully in the task you are doing – you will perform well, regardless of how anxious you are. Furthermore, the energy that you once spent on struggling with fear can now be invested in taking effective action.

ENGAGEMENT AND EXPANSION

In the previous chapter, I talked about the modes of avoidance and automatic pilot, and how the more time we spend in these states, the more we amplify our fear and the greater the negative impact it has on our lives. In this chapter, we're going to look at two alternative modes: engagement and expansion.

You're already familiar with engagement: being fully conscious, living in the present, making contact with the here and now, being fully aware of and connected with your experience. It is the very opposite of autopilot mode.

Similarly, expansion is the opposite of avoidance mode. In expansion mode, rather than trying to get rid of unpleasant feelings, we open up and accommodate them. We make room for them and allow them to come and go in their own good time. It doesn't mean we like them, want them or approve of them; we just stop investing our time and effort in fighting them. And the more space we can give those difficult feelings, the smaller their impact and influence on our lives.

There's an ancient Indian tale that illustrates this point very well. An old Hindu master was fed up with the continual complaints and grumbles of his apprentice. So one day, he asked the young man to fetch him a cup of water and a bowl of salt. When the young man returned, the master said, 'Now tip a handful of salt into the water.' The apprentice did so. The master then swirled the water around in the cup until all the salt had dissolved. 'Now taste it,' he said to the apprentice. The apprentice took a sip and screwed up his face in disgust. 'How does it taste?' asked the master.

'Horrible,' said the apprentice.

The master chuckled. 'Yes, very unpleasant,' he said. 'Now follow me.' They walked down to the edge of a nearby lake, and the master said, 'Now tip a handful of salt into the lake.' The apprentice did so.

The master said, 'Now taste the water from the lake.' The apprentice drank from the lake, and this time he smiled. 'Not so hard to swallow, eh?' said the master. 'This salt is like the inevitable pain of life. In both cases, the amount of salt is the same; but the smaller the container, the greater the bitterness. So when life gives us pain, instead of closing in around it, like this cup, we would do better to enlarge and open, like the lake.'

Lovely story, isn't it? But enough of the chit-chat; now it's time to knuckle down and do it.

NAME YOUR FEELINGS

To handle any strong emotion effectively, we need to NAME it. NAME is an acronym which stands for:

N – Notice
A – Acknowledge
M – Make space
E – Expand awareness

We can use the NAME technique with any difficult emotion, feeling or sensation, but for now we are going to focus solely on fear. Shortly I'll provide you with detailed instructions on how to do it, but first I'll briefly summarize the four different steps.

Note: at first glance, this exercise may seem long and complex, but you'll soon find it's much faster to do it than to read it. And with practice, it gets quicker and easier. Indeed, once you know what you're doing, you can zip through the whole exercise in a few seconds.

Step 1: Notice

Noticing, or paying attention, is at the very heart of mindfulness. Just as the first step in defusion is to notice your thoughts, the first step in expansion is to notice your feelings. So when fear shows up in your body, notice where it is and what it feels like.

Step 2: Acknowledge

Here we use simple self-talk to acknowledge the feeling is present. We silently say to ourselves something like: 'I'm noticing fear', or 'Here's a feeling of fear', or 'Here's fear.' These ways of speaking are unnatural, but they serve a purpose: they help us to separate from the feeling to some degree. Note the difference between 'Here's fear' and 'I'm afraid', or 'I'm noticing fear' versus 'I'm scared'. If we use a phrase such as 'I'm noticing . . .' or 'Here's a feeling of . . .', that helps us to remember we are not our feelings. Our feelings are transient events, continually passing through us and changing like the weather. They do not define who we are or dictate what we do.

Step 3: Make room

Here we 'breathe into' the feeling, psychologically 'open up' and 'make room' for it. When we breathe deeply, it helps to anchor us in the present, and when we 'direct' our breath into and around the feeling, it helps us to drop the struggle with it. The fear is still present, but the more space we give it, the less impact and influence it has on our behaviour.

Step 4: Expand awareness

Having created space for this feeling, we need to re-engage with the world around us. This last stage draws on our engagement skills: we continue to notice the feeling and simultaneously connect with the world around us.

Okay, so that's the summary. Now I'll take you through it in detail. (And if you'd like a voice to guide you, you'll find this exercise on my CD, *Mindfulness Skills: Volume 1,* available as a CD or MP3 from www.thehappinesstrap.co.uk.)

Before we commence, you'll need to dredge up some fear so you've got something to work with. So look back on your values-guided goals from chapter 13, and find one that brings up fear. Now imagine yourself taking some sort of action towards this goal: sitting down to write that book, attending that interview, asking that person for a date, taking out that business loan, enrolling in that course, entering that tournament, going for that audition. Imagine it as vividly as you can: as you take this action, what are you doing with your arms and legs? What can you see, hear, touch, taste and smell? And as you imagine it, see if you can get in touch with your fear.

If you can't tap into your fear merely by thinking about it, then another way is to make a firm commitment: what is one small step you will take today, and a larger step you will take tomorrow, that will get you moving towards your goal? Commit to this right now and chances are fear will show up straight away. And if that still doesn't do the trick, then make your commitment publicly to someone you care about – in person, by phone or by email. That's virtually guaranteed to rev up a fight-or-flight response.

So please do this now, as best you can. Take as long as you need. Then once you've tapped into some fear, let's . . .

NAME IT AND TAME IT!

A quick reminder: NAME stands for notice, acknowledge, make space, and expand awareness. Now, bringing your fear with you so we can work with it, let's get started.

Notice

Many people feel fear most intensely in their throat, chest or abdomen, but you might notice it in *any* part of your body. So take a few seconds to scan yourself from head to toe and notice all the different sensations of fear: what can you feel in your forehead, eyes, jaw, mouth, throat, neck, shoulders, arms, hands, chest, abdomen, pelvis, buttocks, legs and feet?

Now zoom in on the part of your body where the sensations are strongest. Remember, life is like a stage show, and on that stage are all your thoughts, all your feelings, and everything you can see, hear, touch, taste and smell. So shine a bright spotlight on this part of your body, and observe the sensations as if you're a curious scientist.

If your mind starts getting all worked up – 'I hate this feeling', 'I can't stand feeling this way', 'I have to get rid of this feeling' – just thank it for its comments, or let it chatter away like a radio in the background. And the moment you realize you've been hooked, gently acknowledge it, unhook yourself and refocus.

Notice where the feeling starts and stops. Is it moving or still? Is it on the surface of your body, or deep inside? If you drew an outline around it, what shape would it have?

Notice the temperature: is it all the same, or are there hot spots and cold spots?

Notice the different elements within this feeling: pulsation, vibration, throbbing, pressure, temperature and movement.

Again and again, unhook yourself from your thoughts and refocus on those sensations under the spotlight. Observe them with curiosity, as if you were an archaeologist excavating a magnificent ancient temple. Notice every tiny detail. See if you can discover something new that you never previously noticed.

Acknowledge

Now use a few words to acknowledge your feeling by name. Say to yourself, 'I'm noticing fear', or 'Here's a feeling of fear', or 'Here's fear.' (And feel free to substitute other words, such as 'nerves', 'stress' and 'anxiety'.)

Make sure you do this non-judgementally; don't say, 'Oh no, here's this horrible feeling again.' And if you like, you can also remind yourself: 'This is a normal feeling. This is what people feel when they face a challenge.'

Make room

Breathe slowly and deeply. First, breathe *out*. Push all the air out of your lungs – every last bit, until they are completely empty. Then pause for a second with your lungs empty. Then allow them to fill slowly, from the bottom up.

Then once again, breathe out – slowly and steadily, completely emptying your lungs. Then as you breathe in, direct your breath into and around the feeling. (Interpret this instruction any way you like; however you make sense of it is fine. Basically, in some way, sense or imagine your breath flowing into and around the feeling.)

As you breathe into the feeling, imagine that in some magical way a vast space opens up inside you. Instead of closing down this feeling, trying to squash it or crush it, you open up and make room for it.

You don't have to like, want or approve of this feeling. You simply *allow* it to be there. (If you like, you could say to yourself, 'Opening up', 'Making room', or 'Let it be.' Or you could use a longer phrase like, 'I don't like it or want it, but I can make room for it.')

Keep those sensations under the spotlight, observing them with curiosity. And keep breathing into them. Open up little by little, progressively creating more space around the feeling. Remember you're not trying to *get rid* of this feeling; you're simply making room for it!

If you're somewhere private, one thing you can do that often helps is to gently place your hand over the sensations and notice the warmth flowing from your hand into your body. See if you can 'soften up' or 'loosen up' around the feeling. Imagine holding it gently in your hand, as if it's a tiny baby, or a rare butterfly, or a fragile priceless artwork.

Do this for as long as required. Initially it may take you a few minutes to really get that sense of 'making room', but with practice, you can do this in a few seconds. (And if you're struggling with sensations in other parts of your body, then repeat the exercise there.)

Expand awareness

The final step is to expand awareness, so that as well as being aware of your feelings, you are also in touch with the world around you. In other words, you bring up the lights on the whole stage show.

So keep that spotlight on the feeling, and also start to bring up the lights on your body. Sit or stand up straight; notice your arms, legs, head, neck and shoulders. Have a stretch, if you like. Be aware of your body and your fear simultaneously.

Now also bring up the lights on the world around you. Remaining fully aware of your fear and your body, also notice what you can see, hear, touch, taste and smell. This gives you an expansive awareness. Now you can see the whole stage show. Now you can engage in what you are doing.

Remember Sarah, the dancer? Important values she clarified in the domain of work included creativity, courage, persistence, sensuality, connecting with her body, and skilfulness. Her short-term goal was to practise, practise, practise (not only her dance skills, but her defusion skills). Her medium-term goal was to attend more auditions. And her long-term goal was to land a place in a top dance company. When Sarah started attending those auditions, she was terrified. The fear welled up inside her, churning her stomach and squeezing away at her throat. But she practised the NAME technique. She made room for the fear and engaged in her performance. And guess what? She wasn't offered a part at any of the next five auditions. But she didn't give up. She kept practising her routines, she attended classes, and she even saved up for some private tuition. And all the while, she got better and better at defusing from her thoughts of failure and making room for her fear. Finally, on her sixth audition, she landed a supporting role in a popular stage show. She hadn't yet achieved her long-term goal, but she was well on the way and living her values with each and every step of the journey.

TROUBLESHOOTING EXPANSION

If you've never done anything like this exercise before, you'll find it difficult at first. Like any other skill, it needs practice. So I hope you'll practise it several times a day. You can practise this with *any* difficult emotion, not just fear; why not try it with anger, guilt, sadness, impatience or frustration? You can make your practice sessions any length of time you like, from thirty seconds to thirty minutes. With practice, you can do this any time, any place: in a meeting, on the sports field, in bed, at the office, during an argument, on the toilet or in the shower. Indeed, it won't take long before you can run through all four steps in the space of just one deep breath.

There are five main pitfalls to beware of:

a) The hidden agenda

The purpose of expansion is to make room for difficult feelings; to accommodate them, not to evict them. So if you're practising expansion hoping it will get rid of your fear, then you're still in avoidance mode: still trying to avoid or get rid of it. And you've seen already, that won't work. You can't reverse hundreds of millions of years of evolution that have primed you to feel fear when facing a challenge. Trying to get rid of your fear will only amplify it.

b) The illusion of control

At times, you'll do this exercise and find the fear rapidly disappears. When this happens, you'll feel a sense of relief or relaxation. At this point, it's easy to get hooked by the illusion that you've found a clever way to control your feelings: a method for avoiding your fear. But if you start using expansion for that purpose, then clearly you're back into avoidance mode. So if your fear disappears or reduces, then by all means enjoy it, but please don't come to expect it. Regard it as a lucky bonus. If you start to expect it, you'll soon be disappointed.

c) Getting hooked

It's easy for your mind to hook you with unhelpful stories: old favourites like 'I can't do it' or 'It's too hard' or 'I don't have time', or harsh judgements like 'I hate this feeling', or protests like, 'I just want to get rid of it.' You can't stop those thoughts showing up, so don't even try. Just let them come and go like passing cars. (That's why we covered defusion before expansion. If you're getting repeatedly hooked to such an extent that it interferes with expansion, then you'll need to do more work on your defusion skills.)

d) Tolerance

Sometimes people think expansion is about *tolerating* their fear: grinning and bearing it, putting up with it or even resigning themselves to it. This is way off the mark. In expansion, we aim to *allow* our fear. And that doesn't mean we like it, want it or approve of it. It simply means we give it space, and allow it to do its own thing.

To clarify this, imagine that you have an 'avoidance dial' at the back of your mind. This dial goes from zero to ten. When it's on ten, you're in total avoidance mode: you'll do whatever you possibly can to avoid or get rid of this feeling. When it's on zero, you don't like or want this feeling, but you invest absolutely no effort whatsoever in trying to get rid of it. When the dial is at zero, we call this 'acceptance'. When the dial is set around five, we call it 'tolerance'.

Tolerance means you're moving in the direction of acceptance, but you're not there yet. If you sense that you're tolerating rather than accepting, that's okay; it's a good start. Just recognize there's more practice to be done. The experience of fully accepting a feeling, totally dropping the struggle with it, is very different to 'putting up' with it.

e) Forgetting the point

We can easily forget the point of expansion: we make room for difficult feelings in order to live by our values. If we want to live rich and full lives, guided by our values, then we'll have to leave our comfort zones repeatedly – and each time we do, we'll feel fear. Expansion enables us to feel that fear without a struggle, so we can invest our energy in acting on our values.

THE NEXT STEP

In this chapter, you've learned how to *accept* fear:

- Notice it
- Acknowledge it
- Make room for it
- Expand awareness

In the next chapter, you'll discover how to *use* your fear; how to turn it to your advantage. And you'll find it's a bit like . . .

chapter 16

riding a wild stallion

You step on to the front porch of your farmhouse. You feel the warm caress of the morning sun. You stretch your arms wide and breathe in the fresh spring air. Then something on the horizon catches your eye. A shape in the distance, moving very quickly.

You rub your eyes, not quite sure if you are dreaming. But no, it's real. You dash back inside, grab your binoculars, dash back out. Raise them to your eyes. And there it is: a magnificent beast, thundering across the plain, powerful muscles rippling beneath a coat of pure black hair. But it's not one of your own horses. It's a wild stallion. And somehow it has found its way on to your property. So what do you do?

Fear is like a wild stallion. If we know how to harness its energy, we can use it to our advantage. But if we don't know how to handle it, we're in trouble. Imagine approaching a wild stallion without some good horse-wrangling skills: you'd get kicked, bitten or trampled, and waste a lot of time and energy for no useful outcome. On the other hand, if you're a skilled horse-whisperer, then you can approach that horse safely. And over time, if you treat it well, you can build a good relationship with it and eventually ride it.

Now, I have to admit I know absolutely nothing about handling horses. But I do know quite a lot about handling fear. So I'm going to show you how to become a 'fear-whisperer'.

THE ABC OF FEAR-WHISPERING

There's a simple ABC formula for fear-whispering. When fear shows up, we: allow it, befriend it and channel it.

Allow it

Think of that wild stallion racing around. If you ever want to make use of its awesome strength, speed and stamina, you first have to *allow* it to stay on your ranch. And the same goes for fear.

There is a huge amount of energy within our fear. Remember, the fight–or–flight response evolved over hundreds of millions of years to prepare our bodies for action. Fear gives us sharpened reflexes, increased muscle tone, heightened awareness and greater strength. It's like a potent fuel. But we'll never learn how to use that fuel if we're not willing to handle it.

In the previous chapter, you learned how to 'allow' your fear: you notice, acknowledge and make room for it. After allowing, the next step is to . . .

Befriend it

If you want to tame that wild horse, allowing it to stay on your ranch is not enough. You have to build a positive relationship with it; you have to win its trust. How do you do that? Well, from what I've seen in the movies, you approach it cautiously, and talk softly and gently, get closer and closer, and then offer it some tasty food, and if it lets you, stroke its flank, keep talking calmly and sooth-ingly, and show it that you're a friend, not a threat.

Note: we do have to be careful when comparing horses with fear, because horses can seriously injure or even kill you. In con-trast, *fear is totally harmless.* The worst it can do is make us feel very uncomfortable. But that aside, the comparison is useful: if we want to use our fear to our advantage, allowing it isn't enough; we need to befriend it.

Now, at this point your mind may start protesting, 'But I don't *like* this feeling!' Rest assured: you don't have to like it. Let's sup-pose there is a lonely old man in your neighbourhood, and I offer to pay you ten billion dollars to befriend him. And let's suppose this man has some unusual habits; he is prone to angry outbursts of abusive comments, wears filthy clothes and totally neglects his per-sonal hygiene. So you really don't like him. And yet . . . there's ten billion dollars at stake here. Would you make the effort to befriend him, even if you didn't like him? For ten billion dollars, I'm sure you would!

So what about fear? If befriending it helps you to live by your values, achieve your goals, perform at your peak, develop genuine confidence and generally live a richer, fuller, more meaningful life, then will you make the effort, even though you don't like it?

Befriending our fear is just like befriending a person or a horse. Friendliness involves being pleasant, welcoming, affectionate, trust-ing, collaborative and helpful. Does this sound like a tall order? Maybe it is, but I encourage you to give it a try and see what happens.

Be pleasant and welcoming to your fear. It may seem very weird, but try talking to it (making sure to keep a strong sense of humour). You might say, 'Hello, fear. How thoughtful of you to drop by today. Come on in and make yourself at home. What do you want to do today? Oh, you want to give my heart a bit of a workout, do you? Please, do be my guest. See how fast you can get it racing. Oh, you want to chase some butterflies around my stomach? Please, go for it. My house is your house.'

Obviously you wouldn't do something like this in the middle of an interview or a performance, because it would interfere with task-focused attention. But there are plenty of times and places where you could try this, such as in the car, in bed, waiting in queues, during commercial breaks on TV and so on.

Be affectionate towards your fear. If you've got a good imagination, you could imagine shaking fear's hand, inviting it into your body, and slipping your arm warmly around its back. And if you're somewhere private, then you could gently place a hand on the fear – that is, on the part of the body where you feel it most intensely – and 'hold it gently'; let it feel the soothing warmth of your hand.

Be trusting towards your fear. It's not out to get you. Fear evolved for a purpose: to help us handle challenging situations effectively. It alerts us to risks and threats, and readies us for action, should it be necessary. So we'd be in big trouble if we didn't have any.

Be collaborative with your fear. Recognize you're 'playing on the same team'. Don't fight with your fear; it's there to support you. It's a signal; it lets you know you're facing a challenge. So perhaps you could remind yourself, 'This is my brain, alerting me to a challenge; this is my body getting me ready for action.' Regard it as a teammate, not an opponent.

Be helpful towards your fear. Fear evolved to give you strength, speed, focus and stamina. So help it to do its job. Help it to put its energy into something useful, something meaningful, something life-enhancing. In other words . . .

Channel it

Cast your mind back once more to that wild stallion. You've allowed it to stay and befriended it. Now what? Now you want to use it to your benefit; to saddle it up and ride it.

And so it is with fear. You've allowed it, befriended it – now use it. Take a moment to notice how much energy it gives you: all that adrenaline flowing through your system. Your whole body is geared up for action. As I mentioned earlier, many successful athletes, businesspeople and stage performers don't use the word 'fear' to describe those feelings they have when facing a challenge. They often talk instead of being 'revved', 'pumped', 'juiced', 'wired' or 'amped'. These terms all acknowledge the energizing aspects of the fight-or-flight response.

So ask yourself, 'How can I make use of all this energy? What values-guided activities can I channel it into?'

Of course, there are situations where you *can't* channel your fear into something useful. For example, if you're out on a first date, chatting away in a quiet bar or restaurant, there's not much you can do with all that energy. In such an instance, you just make room for it and engage fully in the present.

However, there are plenty of times when you *can* make good use of your energy. For example, if you're playing sport, being physically active or giving some sort of performance, then you can channel all this 'fear energy' into it.

Reminding yourself to use your fear can make a huge difference at times. Over the past few years, I've been giving talks and workshops in Australia, the US and Europe, to audiences varying in size from half a dozen to several thousand. Do I feel confident about doing this? Well, most of the time, yes I do. I certainly *didn't* feel confident when I first started, but now I've had so much practice that I generally do. However, when I'm speaking on a new topic, or running a brand-new type of workshop, I definitely do *not* feel confident. (Nor do I expect to, until I've done it over and over.) But I do act with confidence: I get up on stage, give the speech or workshop and engage fully in the task.

Now here's the thing: regardless of whether or not I feel confident, I always feel fear. If that surprises you, let me remind you of some basic human biology: when we're facing a genuine challenge, we're going to have a fight-or-flight response. So no matter how confident we are at doing something, if the situation is challenging, we'll feel fear. You may recall this rule:

Rule 2: Genuine confidence is not the absence of fear; it is a transformed relationship *with fear.*

Thus, before I start my talk or workshop, I make room for my fear, take a deep breath, and say to myself, 'Okay! Here we go! Let's put this energy into action!' The fear is still there, but my relationship with it has transformed. Now it's not just something I need to make room for in order to get on with my life. Now it's something useful in its own right. It's a potent fuel; a burst of energy that revs me up, gets me buzzing and enhances my performance.

And you can do the same thing in your life. Remind yourself regularly to channel your fear and notice the difference it makes when you do so. It may take a while to get the hang of this, but when you do, it makes a huge difference. Indeed, over time, you may find yourself using words like 'revved', 'pumped' and 'amped', instead of 'fear' and 'anxiety'. And if there's nothing for you to channel your fear into, then make room for it and engage fully in whatever you are doing.

WHERE TO NEXT?

This brings us to the end of part 4 of the book. In the fifth and final part, we're going to tie it all together: values, goals, actions, defusion, engagement and expansion. And we'll also look at self-motivation, overcoming obstacles, and the keys to peak performance. For now, we'll finish up with one more rule for winning the confidence game:

Rule 8: Don't fight your fear; allow it, befriend it and channel it.

part five

playing the game

chapter 17

throw off the bowlines

As Joe Simpson dragged himself back to base camp, snow-blind, frozen, starving and dehydrated, fingers ravaged by frostbite, his shattered leg firing volleys of agonizing pain, what kept him going?

It wasn't positive thinking, self-hypnosis or asking the universe to provide. What kept him going were his values of commitment, courage, persistence and self-preservation. Joe knew that the odds of making it back alive were millions to one. His two climbing companions believed he was dead, so there would be no reason at all for them to hang around at base camp, waiting for him. Joe knew it would take him at least a couple of days to get back there, and by then it would almost certainly be deserted – if he even made it that far. The chances were that he would die before he got back, from exposure and exhaustion.

But to Joe, the idea of giving up was far worse than the alternative of trying and failing. He knew there was a chance, just a tiny, ever-so-improbable chance, that maybe, just maybe, his companions would still be there when he arrived; maybe he *would* actually make it.

He knew this chance was ridiculously small; so improbable that he tried hard not to even think about it. But what he did think about was this: if he gave up trying, if he lay down and surrendered to his fate, then he would definitely die. At least while he kept moving, he had a chance. So rather than choose certain death, he chose survival; rather than choose to quit, he chose commitment; rather than choose defeat, he chose persistence; rather than choose despair, he chose courage. And as he dragged himself through that bleak, barren landscape of snow and ice, feeling hopeless and scared, he lived his values every step of the way: courage, commitment, persistence and self-preservation; being true to himself; giving it everything he had; fighting to the bitter end.

VALUES AREN'T ENOUGH

Joe Simpson's values were vitally important; they inspired him to keep on going, and guided the actions he took. But values aren't enough for genuine confidence or peak performance. Remember, our values are like a compass: a compass can give us direction, but it can't transport us. Our journey only begins when we start taking action. So we use our values to set goals, then we break our goals down into actions. And as we take action, we do so mindfully, engaging fully in the task. Joe's story illustrates this process very well.

Consider values and goals. Values are what we want to stand for; how we want to behave on an ongoing basis. Goals are what we want to have, get or achieve. Joe Simpson's *goal* was to reach base camp. His values were courage, self-preservation, commitment and doing his best. He knew the chances were high that he'd fail at his *goal* – however, with every excruciating step, he lived his *values*.

Early on in his journey, when Joe looked off into the distance and saw how far he had to go, he felt despair. It was too far, too hard, too painful. He had no food or water. He wasn't strong enough to do it. So he stopped focusing on the long-term goal and instead set himself short-term goals: get to the bottom of this slope; get to the other side of that ice bridge; dig a snow hole to sleep in. At times, he even set himself time limits: half an hour to hop to that pillar of rock; three hours to crawl his way to the lake.

Each of those short-term goals required action. He wouldn't get anywhere if he didn't move his arms and legs. Those actions weren't easy: every crawl, hop and twist racked him with pain. And when he fell, he would sometimes pass out from the agony. Hardly surprising, then, that at times Joe was overwhelmed by his challenge. He would give up trying and lie down in the snow, ready to die. However, after a while, he always got back up again. And again and again and again, living his values and engaging fully in the task.

In *Touching the Void*, Simpson never mentions the word 'mindfulness', but he frequently describes the concept in his own words. For example, early on in his journey, he had to make his way up steep slopes covered in snow. So he would plant his axes in the snow, press his arms down hard for extra thrust, then hop off on his good leg and heave up his shattered leg behind him.

Incredibly, he managed to engage fully in this routine, in an awe-inspiring example of task-focused attention. Here's how he describes it: 'The flares of pain became merged into the routine and I paid less attention to them, concentrating solely on the patterns.' It was an incredible exertion, and despite the sub-zero temperature, he was dripping with sweat. But he didn't stop. And as he kept moving, his agonizing pain became one with his physical efforts. Before long, he was so engaged in the activity, he lost all track of time. In his own words: 'Time passed unnoticed as I became absorbed with the patterns of hopping and digging.'

Now, although Joe's circumstances were extreme, and hopefully we will never experience anything like them, there are at least six lessons we can learn from his amazing story.

SIX LESSONS WE CAN LEARN FROM JOE SIMPSON

Lesson 1: When we face major challenges in life, if we move forward guided by our values, we will feel a sense of meaning and purpose. And we will find satisfaction in knowing we are doing what really matters to us. On the other hand, when we 'give up' and shrink from our challenges, we feel like our lives are slipping away. As a general rule, when we choose to give up, to stop pursuing what is truly important in life, that is usually worse than the alternative of trying and failing.

Is your mind protesting? Is it trying to disprove my last comment? Our minds are very clever, and I'm willing to bet they can come up with examples where we would be better off giving up on our goals than pursuing them. And rightly so, because what I said is a generalization, not a hard-and-fast rule for all occasions. As a *general rule*, to be held lightly and flexibly, giving up on doing what matters will be worse, in terms of health, wellbeing and life satisfaction, than pursuing what matters and failing. As the great author Mark Twain put it: 'Twenty years from now you will be more disappointed by the things that you didn't do than by the ones you did do. So throw off the bowlines. Sail away from the safe harbour. Catch the trade winds in your sails. Explore. Dream. Discover.'

Lesson 2: Even when we think a goal is impossible, we can still keep moving towards it. We don't have to *believe* that we will achieve it; we just have to take action. Against all the odds, Joe achieved his goal. Most people in his situation would never have made it. That's the way life goes: sometimes we will achieve our goals and sometimes we won't. And like it or not, we have no way of knowing what the outcome will be. At times we will be absolutely convinced that we will succeed, but we will fail. At other times we'll be sure that we're going to fail, and then we succeed. Many motivational gurus claim that you must be certain of success in order to move forward; that you must completely believe that you will achieve your goals. Joe Simpson's story proves this is not the case.

Lesson 3: As long as we keep moving forward, every little step counts. Each and every step is an important part of the journey.

Lesson 4: Moving in a meaningful direction often gives rise to uncomfortable thoughts, feelings and sensations. Fortunately, we're not talking about the agonizing pain and fear of death that Joe Simpson had to endure; but we will all commonly feel fear, self-doubt and anxiety as we act on our values, and if we play a sport or do other physical pursuits, then painful sensations are also going to arise as we tax our muscles. So if we want to achieve our most important goals in life, we'd better learn to make room for discomfort.

Lesson 5: When the going gets tough, the tough get mindful. If we wish to act effectively in challenging situations, we need to engage fully in what we are doing. We can't stop those difficult thoughts and feelings from arising, but we can stop investing our energy in struggling with them, and instead focus on the task at hand. Through engaging fully in his hopping, Joe was able to keep going despite unimaginable pain. If he had fused with all his thoughts of hopelessness, he'd never have made it.

Lesson 6: At times, we will all give up, as Joe Simpson did each time he lay down in the snow ready to die. Commitment doesn't mean we never give up or go off track. Commitment means that when we *do* give up or go off track, we pick ourselves up, dust ourselves down, and get back on track again! In the words of the great Chinese philosopher Confucius: 'Our greatest glory is not in never falling, but in rising every time we fall.'

OVER TO YOU

So that's Joe Simpson's story; what's yours going to be? What daring adventures are you going to have? What new frontiers are you going to explore? What important risks are you going to take? You don't have to go climbing mountains, hunting fossils or defying racist regimes. Daring adventures can include almost anything: going on a blind date, sitting down at a desk to write that book, enrolling in a course, giving that speech, taking that dance class, picking up that paintbrush, going for that interview, entering that tournament or making that big pitch. A daring adventure for Raj was setting up his new restaurant. For Sarah, it was dancing. For Claire, it was expanding her social life. For Cleo, it was dating guys. And for Seb, it was making love to his wife again.

To create your own daring adventure is very simple. It only requires five basic steps.

Step 1: Pick a domain of life

Choose one domain of life to work on first: love, work, or play. (It's important to pick only one, as if you try to work on all three simultaneously, you'll probably get overwhelmed; over time, you can focus on the others.)

Step 2: Clarify values

Take a couple of minutes to reflect on your values within this domain of life: What sort of character do you want to build? What personal qualities do you want to develop? What do you want to stand for?

Step 3: Set goals
Now use these values to set yourself some goals. What are some short-term goals you can aim for in the next few days and weeks? What are some medium-term goals for the next few weeks and months? What are some long-term goals for the ensuing months and years?

Step 4: Specify actions
Choose an important short-term goal. What actions are necessary to achieve it? What's the very first step? What's the simplest, easiest thing you could do to make a start today – no matter how small a step it might be?

Step 5: Get moving
Okay, you know what you need to do, so now get moving! And as you do, remember to act mindfully: unhook yourself from unhelpful stories, make room for uncomfortable feelings, and engage fully in whatever task you are doing.

Here's how Seb did it. The domain of life that he focused on first was his marriage. Some important values he clarified were: being loving, affectionate, sensual and intimate. His long-term goal was to resume regular sexual intercourse with his wife. His short-term goal was simply to initiate physical affection. His medium-term goal was to gradually progress through increasingly intimate physical activities, such as massage, mutual masturbation and oral sex, until he was ready to attempt intercourse again.

The first small action Seb took was to cuddle his wife in bed; to hold her firmly in his arms. This was a significant step out of his comfort zone. For the last few years, he'd always kept well over to his side of the bed, afraid to cuddle his wife for fear that one thing might lead to another. Seb defused from all his worries, made room for the fear in his stomach, chest and neck, and engaged fully in the cuddle, noticing the warm and pleasant sensations that arose from their intertwined bodies. In this manner, little by little, step by step, Seb and his wife gradually resumed their sex life. It took about four months before they had intercourse, but they both said it was well worth the wait!

So now it's your turn. What's your daring adventure going to be?

I STILL DON'T HAVE ENOUGH CONFIDENCE!

If your mind is protesting that you still don't have the confidence to start taking action, then thank it kindly and remember the golden rule:

The actions of confidence come first; the feelings of confidence come later.

If you're waiting for the feelings of confidence before you start your daring adventure, you'll be waiting forever. The trick is to embark on your adventure and travel mindfully, guided by your values, even if you don't feel the way you'd prefer to. This would be an example of *acting* with confidence.

Also keep in mind that you now have all the tools you need to effectively address the five main causes of low self-confidence:

1. **Excessive expectations:** You can deal with this via defusion and engagement. Unhook yourself from all those perfectionist demands and engage fully in the task at hand.

2. **Harsh self-judgement:** Again, defusion and engagement are the keys. Develop self-acceptance by

unhooking yourself from all self-judgements (both positive and negative). Defuse from your mind's commentary on your performance and engage fully in what you're doing.

3. **Preoccupation with fear:** This requires expansion, defusion and engagement. Make room for feelings of fear; unhook yourself from stories of failure, rejection and disaster; and engage fully in whatever task you are completing.

4. **Lack of experience:** This requires values, expansion and committed action. We only get experience in doing things if we step out of our comfort zones and do them. So connect with your values, make room for fear and get moving.

5. **Lack of skills:** This too requires values, expansion and committed action. Use values such as persistence, dedication or 'giving it your best' to motivate yourself. Make room for the discomfort involved – which could be anything from boredom and frustration to fear or physical pain – and do what needs to be done to improve those skills. And make sure you're working on the *right* skills, the ones that can really make a difference. Many athletes and businesspeople kid themselves: they work hard at the skills that come most easily, but avoid practising the more challenging skills that could take their performance to the next level.

In the points above, I've highlighted the skills most relevant to the issue, but really, everything we've covered in this book applies in each and every case. Whatever is interfering with our confidence, the solution lies in mindfulness, values and action: defuse from unhelpful thoughts, expand around difficult feelings, take action guided by our values, and engage fully in whatever we are doing.

We can remember this with the acronym ACT:

A – Accept your thoughts and feelings
C – Choose a valued direction
T – Take action mindfully

So there you have it: everything you need to start your daring adventure and develop genuine confidence along the way. And by 'genuine confidence', I mean the ability to act on your values, regardless of how you are feeling: to trust and rely on yourself to do what matters, even if you feel terrified!

Now pause for ten seconds, and notice what your mind is saying.

***

If you were hoping for a magic wand to control your feelings, then your mind is probably making some sort of protest, feeling annoyed at my definition of 'genuine confidence'. And there's nothing abnormal in that. Our minds like to get their own way, and when that doesn't happen, they like to complain. So once again, thank your mind for its input and consider the question below.

THE BIG CHOICE
Suppose I could give you a choice about how to live your life. There are two options:

Option one: for the rest of your life, you only take action to do the things that are really important to you if you are in the mood, psyched up and feeling good. In other words, you spend the rest of your days on this planet at the mercy of your emotions. If you're 'in the mood' or you feel good, then you do the things that make your life work. But if your mood drops or you don't feel good, then you give up doing the things that truly matter, and put your life on hold until such time as you feel good, positive or inspired again.

Option two: for the rest of your life, you take action to do the things that are really important to you, whether you are 'in the mood' or not. Whether you feel good or bad, energetic or tired, optimistic or pessimistic, calm or anxious, relaxed or fearful, inspired or uninspired, you continue to take action; you keep doing what truly matters to you. Instead of going through life at the mercy of your emotions, you can behave like the person you want to be and do the things you want to do, even if you're tired or anxious, or you don't feel like it.

Which do you choose?

If you choose option one, you're setting yourself up for a life of struggle: investing more and more of your time, effort and money in trying to control your feelings, while all the time missing out on doing what matters.

If you choose option two, it's a recipe for success and fulfilment. Look closely at the people you consider most successful in life, and you'll find this is the option they have chosen. Read a few biographies of top athletes, artists, performers, politicians or businesspeople, and this will soon become crystal clear. What characterizes these people is *not* that they were always feeling good, positive, optimistic, inspired, 'psyched up' or in the mood. What characterizes them is their willingness to persist through thick and thin, through ups and downs, through trials and tribulations. Yes, even when they felt afraid, tired, hopeless or miserable, they continued to act on their values!

There's a lovely paradox in choosing the second option. When we let go of trying to control our feelings, and instead start acting on our values and engaging fully in whatever we are doing, then pleasant feelings often show up for the ride. We are likely to feel healthier, happier and calmer. But please note: this is a by-product of values-based living; a lovely bonus, but not the main aim. The aim of mindful, values-based living is to create a rich, full and meaningful life, while accepting the pain that goes with it.

Assuming you chose option two, it's time to get moving. You already know the drill: pick a domain; clarify your values; set some goals; take action; engage fully in what you do. So take a moment to clarify your next step and then take action.

And if you're still not moving after that pep talk, then it's time to clarify . . .

chapter 18

what's stopping you?

The queue seems to stretch on for ever: a line of human figures, trailing off into the distance, until they are nothing but tiny black dots on the horizon.

To the left of the queue, there's a stranded bus, the passengers staring lifelessly out of the windows. In front of the bus, there's a long couch on which strangely garbed humans and a bizarre bird sit twiddling their thumbs. Everywhere you look, people are waiting: a man slumped at his desk, gazing desperately at the clock; a young girl watching a pot that never boils; an important-looking official staring at a phone that doesn't ring.

Where is this? It is The Waiting Place, as illustrated in Dr Seuss's marvellous book, *Oh, the Places You'll Go!* In his unique style, Dr Seuss describes how this 'most useless place' is full of people 'just waiting'. They are waiting for anything and everything: for trains, buses and planes; for changes in the weather; for fish to bite, mail to arrive or hair to grow. They have put their lives on hold, unwilling to move on until they have received what they are waiting for. No wonder they all look so miserable.

We all get bogged down in The Waiting Place at times: waiting until we're in the mood, or we feel confident, or the time is right, before we start doing what really matters to us. And that's only natural. After all, we're human beings, not superheroes. It'd be fantastic if there were some magic button we could push that just got us out there, strutting our stuff. But it's not that easy.

Don't get me wrong – I've seen many people make rapid and dramatic progress using the principles in this book. All I'm saying is that everyone gets stuck at times; even the most successful politicians, musicians, actors, artists, athletes and business leaders go through periods where they get bogged down in The Waiting Place. And when it happens, beating ourselves up about it doesn't help. That would just make us *even more* stuck and miserable. No, if we want to get out of this place, the first thing we need to know is what's keeping us there.

WHAT KEEPS US STUCK?

What holds us back? What stops us from acting on our values? The answer is: FEAR. No, not fear, but FEAR, an acronym that stands for:

F – Fusion
E – Excessive goals
A – Avoidance of discomfort
R – Remoteness from values

Let's look at each of these in turn.

Fusion

Our minds have developed so many clever ways to hook us, it's impossible to cover them all in a book of this length. Still, we've identified some of the most common ones, including perfection-ism, self-judgement, predicting the worst, rehashing old failures, and telling ourselves 'I can't do it' and 'I'm not good enough.' The mind is like a reason–giving machine, and the bigger the challenge we face, the longer the list of reasons it will crank out: why we can't do it, shouldn't do it, or shouldn't have to do it. None of these thoughts are problematic as long as we're defused from them. But if we *fuse* with them, they turn into major obstacles.

So any time you're stuck, ask yourself: 'What story am I fusing with?'

Excessive goals

If your goal exceeds your resources, you will fail. If you want to climb Mount Everest, you need a massive number of resources: you need lots of time, lots of money, excellent physical health, excellent climbing skills and lots of social support. Without these resources, forget it. So ask yourself, 'Is this goal in some way excessive? Am I trying to do too much, too soon?'

Avoidance of discomfort

Step out of your comfort zone and what have you got? Discomfort. This can take many different forms, but by far the most common are fear, anxiety, 'nerves', self-doubt and insecurity. (Of course, discomfort *can* include every private experience a human EMITS: emotions, memories, images, thoughts and sensations.) If you're not willing to make room for discomfort, then you're well and truly stuck in The Waiting Place. Waiting, waiting, waiting; des-perately hoping that if you just wait long enough, the 'right' thoughts and feelings will show up. So ask yourself, 'What thoughts and feelings am I trying to avoid or get rid of? What sort of dis-comfort am I struggling with?'

Remoteness from values

Why would we bother to step out of our comfort zones and do something that's likely to bring up uncomfortable thoughts and feelings? Our values provide the motivation. So if we haven't clarified them, or we've lost touch with them, then we can easily get stuck; after all, what's the point of doing something uncomfortable unless it enriches our lives in the long term? So when you're stuck, ask yourself, 'What values am I forgetting, neglecting, or acting inconsistently with?'

Using the FEAR acronym, we can turn 'getting stuck' to our advantage: it becomes an opportunity to develop insight and self-awareness, and identify our mental obstacles. And once we have that information, we can figure out . . .

HOW TO GET UNSTUCK

The antidote to FEAR is to DARE. Yes, DARE is another acronym, which stands for:

D – Defusion
A – Acceptance of discomfort
R – Realistic goals
E – Embracing values

Defusion

Once you know what's hooking you, you can notice it, name it and neutralize it. Thank your mind for its comments. Name the story. Let Radio Triple F play on in the background. Put your thoughts on leaves, or sing them to the tune of your choice. Catch your mind in the act: 'Aha! Reason-giving again!' or 'Aha! The "I can't do it" story!' Engage fully in what you are doing, and let your thoughts come and go like passing cars.

Acceptance of discomfort

In order to do what matters, are you willing to make room for discomfort? Are you willing to make room for the voice in your head that says, 'I can't do it. I'll fail'? Are you willing to make room for a knot in your stomach, a racing heart and sweaty hands? Are you willing to make room for strong emotions such as fear and anger? Are you willing to make room for painful memories, or scary predictions of the future? If not, then you're well and truly stuck inside the comfort zone. In which case, it may help you to think about it like this: There is no such thing as a pain-free life. But we do have some choice about the *type* of pain we experience: we can choose the pain of stagnation, or we can choose the pain of growth.

If we continue to grow, to expand our comfort zones, to try out new things, to explore new horizons, to turn our lives into daring adventures, then we will experience the pain of growth. The pain of growth includes plenty of fear: fear of failure, fear of rejection, fear of making mistakes, fear of wasting time, fear of losing money, fear of reprisal, fear of embarrassment and so on. But we will be feeling that pain in the service of a great adventure: making room for it as we maximize our potential. This pain is accompanied by a sense of vitality, meaning and purpose; a sense of personal growth and living life to the full.

The alternative is to choose the pain of stagnation; of living our lives inside the comfort zone. And that choice comes with huge costs. Personally, I think we really shouldn't call it 'the comfort zone', as that makes it sound like a like a cosy café or a health and beauty spa, rather than a place that drains our lives away. Here are some better names for it: 'the stuck zone', 'the stagnant zone', 'the zombie zone', 'the life half-lived zone', 'the missing out zone', 'the restricted life zone', 'the lost opportunity zone', 'the wasted time zone', 'the same old shit zone', 'the life on hold zone'. (Or maybe just The Waiting Place.) Much like the pain of growth, the pain of stagnation includes plenty of fear: fear of failure, fear of rejection, fear of making mistakes, fear of reprisal, fear of embarrassment, fear of missing out, fear of wasting your life. But there is no vitality, meaning or purpose; no sense of adventure; no personal growth.

So which sort of pain will you choose? Are you willing to accept your discomfort in order to live a full life? If so, what sensations will you need to make room for in your body, and what words and pictures will you need to make room for in your head?

Realistic goals

If your goal exceeds your resources, then you have two options. One option is to put this goal on hold temporarily and set a new goal to find the necessary resources. Thus, if the resource you need is time, then the new goal is to rearrange your schedule: what are you willing to give up or scale back in order to free up time? If the resource you require is physical health, then what can you do to improve it? If it's money you're lacking, then how can you earn, save or borrow it? If it's social support you need, then your new goal is to build up a social network. And if the issue is a deficit in your skills, then your new goal is to work on developing them. Once you have the necessary resources, you can return to the original goal.

The second option is to scale down the goal to fit the resources available: in other words to make it smaller, easier or simpler.

Of course, when it comes to making our goals more realistic, we do have to be careful, because our minds are quick to tell us what we're incapable of. If Joe Simpson had fused with his mind's story that he lacked the resources necessary to achieve his goal, he'd have given up and died in that snowy wasteland. So Joe was very smart. His big goal, getting back to base camp, was too overwhelming for him to contemplate seriously; he didn't believe he had the resources (food, water, equipment, strength and time) to achieve it. On the other hand, he didn't want to give up on it, as that would have spelled certain death. So he scaled it down into a series of much smaller goals – hop to the end of this slope, crawl over to that boulder, and so on – each of which he had the resources to achieve.

This is a good basic strategy whenever we think a goal is impossible: break it down into smaller ones. It's like that old joke – Question: 'How do you eat an elephant?' Answer: 'One mouthful at a time.' For example, if I sat down at my desk, and my goal was 'to write a book', I'd feel overwhelmed by the size of the task. Of course, 'writing a book' *is* my big goal – but when I haven't yet written so much as a single word, achieving it seems almost impossible. So when I sit down at my desk, my goal is usually 'to write for one hour', or perhaps two or three hours. These smaller goals feel much more achievable. Even if I sit at my computer for one hour, and in that time I only write fifty words, and they're all crap, then I've still achieved my goal of writing for an hour. And as hour builds upon hour, and I edit and rewrite and edit some more and rewrite yet again, the book gradually gets completed.

So a useful question to ask ourselves, whenever a goal seems to exceed our resources, is this: 'What's the smallest, simplest, easiest little step I could take in the next twenty-four hours that would take me a tiny bit closer to achieving it?'

Embracing values

What matters to you in the big picture? What sort of life do you want to live? What sort of person do you want to be? What do you want to stand for? Get in touch with these values; reflect on them and let them guide you. When the going gets tough, remind yourself what you're standing for; reflect on the values you're living by.

If these values are important to you, are you willing to act on them? And if so, what are some simple actions you can take? (And if you discover that the goals you've set are not truly aligned with your core values, change them!)

MYTH-BUSTING TIME AGAIN

One of the most unhelpful myths you'll encounter in the world of popular motivation and self-development is this one: you must absolutely believe, 100 per cent, that you will achieve your goal. People who play by this rule really are setting themselves up for a struggle. Why? Because the bigger and more challenging the goal is, the harder it is for most people to believe *100 per cent* that they will achieve it; doubts are commonplace, even amongst the most successful people on the planet. Plus, if someone is actually egotistical or arrogant enough to go through life totally believing that they will succeed at every important goal they set, sooner or later they will get a big shock, because everybody, no matter how talented and driven they are, will fail at times. (Chapter 20 is entirely devoted to this issue.)

Fortunately, you do not have to believe completely that you'll win the contract in order to put in your proposal. You do not have to believe completely that the answer will be yes in order to ask someone out on a date. You do not have to believe completely that you will win the competition in order to enter. All you need do is to acknowledge *there's a possibility* – even if it's tiny. And once you've acknowledged it's possible, you can play by this rule: *Don't obsess about the outcome; get passionate about the process.*

THE REALITY GAP

Whenever there's a large 'reality gap' – by which I mean a gap between the reality we want and the reality we've got – painful feelings will arise. And the larger that reality gap, the greater the pain. A small reality gap may give rise to feelings of disappointment, frustration, anxiety, regret, boredom, guilt or impatience. An enormous reality gap may give rise to despair, angst, rage or terror.

Some of the most painful reality gaps occur when important life goals become truly impossible. For example, once you have a prison record or a history of severe mental illness, there are all sorts of professions which you become permanently barred from entering. Likewise, if you're suffering from an incurable, debilitating illness or you're severely disabled, there are all sorts of activities that are no longer possible – at least, with the science of today.

This is where mindfulness and values come to our aid. We can open up and make room for all those painful feelings, acknowledge that it hurts like hell, and be kind and compassionate to ourselves. We can then ask ourselves: 'What do I want to stand for in the face of this gap?' No matter how much pain we are in, we have a choice to make: we can stand for giving up on life, or we can stand for living by our values. No prizes for guessing which choice gives us the greatest sense of fulfilment and vitality.

On 28 April 1996, thirty-five people were slaughtered in Tasmania during a horrific shooting spree dubbed the 'Port Arthur Massacre'. A couple of years ago I went to an inspiring and heart-rending talk by Walter Mikac, whose wife and two young daughters were killed on that fateful day. There was not a dry eye in the house as he talked about the horrors he'd had to endure. And we were all deeply inspired by Walter's message: he knew it was impossible for him to change the past or bring his family back from the dead – but he desperately wanted to create something positive from the devastation. And so he did. He not only played a major role in tightening Australia's gun laws, but he established a thriving children's charity, the Alannah and Madeline Foundation (named after his daughters), which provides support to child victims of violence.

This is a shining example of living by one's values in the face of a truly enormous reality gap. So if, for one reason or another, our goal truly is impossible, then let's acknowledge that, make room for the pain, and simultaneously get in touch with our values. We could ask ourselves, 'Ten years from now, when I look back on this period in my life, what would I like to say that I stood for; what values did I live by, in the face of that reality gap?' We can then use those values to set some new and different goals – and take our pain with us as we pursue them.

IN AND OUT OF THE COMFORT ZONE

Again and again and again throughout our lives, we're going to get stuck in our comfort zones. Sometimes we'll only stay there briefly. Sometimes we'll get stuck there for ages. But although we'll never be perfect, we can improve. We can get quicker at recognizing when we're stuck, quicker at getting ourselves unstuck, and better at staying on track for longer stretches. The FEAR and DARE acronyms will help you to do this. So I encourage you to memorize them. You could even write them on a card, and carry them around in your wallet. Refer to them repeatedly until you have internalized them. And of course, don't just intellectualize them; put them into action. Doing this will pay huge dividends, not least of which is avoiding . . .

chapter 19

the motivation trap

Has anyone ever told you they can do something that is humanly impossible? I regularly work with clients who make such claims. Here's what they typically say: 'I want to do it, but I have no motivation.'

To 'have no motivation' is quite simply impossible. Unless you're dead, that is. Every action we take has some underlying motivation; it is always intended to achieve something. Whether we're adjusting our position in a chair, eating a piece of toast, shooing away a fly, riding a bike, giving a speech, digging for fossils, commenting on the weather, asking someone to pass the salt, cancelling a social event, ringing in sick, putting off going to the gym or flaking out on the couch, there is always some underlying purpose or intention to our actions; there is always some motivation, even if we are not consciously aware of it.

In fact, we always have multiple motivations, and we can never consciously know every single influence on our behaviour. But we can get good at recognizing the main motivation underlying whatever we're doing.

Before we go any further, let's clarify the meaning of the word: 'motivation' is the desire to do something. And that's *all* it is. It's not some magical drug that gives us the power to do whatever we want; it's simply the desire to do it. To illustrate the point, here's a conversation I had with one of my clients. Let's call him Nate. Nate was a keen football player, but he was about to lose his place on the team because he wasn't turning up for his training sessions. We had previously identified some of Nate's key values as keeping fit, honing his skills, supporting his teammates and giving his best to the game.

Russ: So what's stopping you from going along to the sessions?

Nate: I've just got no motivation.

Russ: Okay, so what are you doing instead of going to training?

Nate: Well, you know, by the time I get home from work, I'm just so tired. I can't be bothered doing anything.

Russ: So what do you do?

Nate: I guess I usually crash on the couch and watch TV.

Russ: So suppose I rang you one evening while you were crashed on the couch and I said, 'Hey, Nate, get your butt off that couch and go to training', what would you say to me?'

Nate: I'd say 'Get f★★★ed!'

Russ: Fair enough. But once you'd calmed down, and assuming you didn't hang up on me, what reason would you give me for opting out of training?

Nate: I'm too tired.

Russ: You'd rather watch TV?

Nate: Yeah.

Russ: So your desire to crash on the couch and watch TV is greater than your desire to go to training?

Nate: [sounding defensive] I want to go, I'm just too tired.

Russ: I'm sorry if you perceive my words as critical. My aim here is not to criticize you. It is purely to give you a more helpful way of looking at your own behaviour so you can learn from it and change it – if that's important to you. Is that okay with you?

Nate: Sure.

Russ: So let's think about this for a moment. The first thing to remember is that our behaviour always serves a purpose. So what purpose is served by crashing on the couch and watching TV, instead of going to training?

Nate: It's relaxing, I guess.

Russ: So in the short term it makes you feel good and helps you avoid the discomfort of going to training?

Nate: Yes.

Russ: But unfortunately, in the long term, it's not helping you to live the life you want. Your skills are getting rusty, your fitness level is dropping, and you're in danger of being kicked off the team.

Nate: Yes.

Russ: So can we say it like this: it's not that you have no motivation. It's simply that your motivation to avoid discomfort and do what feels good in the short term is triumphing over your motivation to keep fit, hone your skills, support your teammates and give your best to the game?

Nate: [pause] Okay. I hadn't seen it that way, but yes, I would agree with that.

Russ: So here's the thing. I'm going to share with you my experience, and I want you to see if it fits with yours. If not, that's fine; you don't have to agree with me. But in my experience, when someone says 'I don't have the motivation' what they really mean is, 'I have a desire to do it, and it is important to me – but I'm not willing to take action unless I feel good, happy, positive, inspired, energized, confident, or "in the mood". As long as I feel tired, sleepy, lazy, anxious, fearful, unconfident or "not in the mood", then I'm not going to do it.' I'm wondering if you can relate to that at all?

Nate: [long pause] Well I don't like to admit it, but . . . yes, that's about right.

MOTIVATION VS COMMITMENT

Nate, like most people, understands motivation to be primarily a feeling. If we feel good about doing something – if we're positive, excited, enthusiastic, revved up or inspired – then we say we 'feel motivated'. And if we don't have those pleasant feelings, then we say we're 'unmotivated' or we've 'got no motivation'. Unfortunately, if we equate motivation with a feeling, we will soon get stuck. Why? Because it pulls us back into the trap of trying to get the right feelings *before* we take action. And as we know, that's a sure-fire way to get bogged down in The Waiting Place.

However, once we recognize that motivation simply means desire, we're in a much better space for changing our behaviour; we can quickly assess our competing desires and recognize what is motivating the choices we make. And in particular, we want to distinguish between the desire to avoid discomfort and the desire to act on our values. These motivations will often pull us in wildly different directions – and the avoidance-driven life is far less rewarding than the values-driven life.

Now, we can't eliminate our desire to avoid discomfort; it's a basic human instinct. But we can make room for it and choose to act on our values instead. To do this requires a major change in our mindset: we need to shift the emphasis from 'motivation' to 'commitment'.

It's easiest to explain this with an example. Since I became a published author, scores of people have come up to me and told me they want to write books. However, very, very few of them ever actually sit down and write one. Lack of motivation is not the problem: they all have the desire to write. What's missing is the commitment: they are not willing to do what is required.

Almost always, what's stopping them is the confidence gap: they're waiting until the day they feel confident before they're willing to take action. And as you know, life doesn't work that way. At this point in the book, you probably know the golden rule off by heart, but just for good measure here it is again: *The actions of confidence come first; the feelings of confidence come later.*

The 'motivation gap' is very similar to the confidence gap: we wait until we feel motivated before we commit to action. Fortunately, we can tweak the golden rule to help us escape: *Committed action comes first; feeling motivated comes later.*

I've experienced the truth of this many, many times while writing this book. At the start of a session I usually have to force myself to write. I make my fingers hit the keypads and I push out the words, one by one. My jaw is tense, I have knots in my stomach, and my mind screams 'This is utter crap!' The temptation to quit is almost irresistible; there are so many other things I could do that would give me some short-term pleasure and help me avoid this discomfort. But I come back to my values – creativity, self-expression, helping others, facing my challenges, improving my ability to communicate – and I commit to doing the writing. And at times, the entire session is a gruelling slog. That's when I empathise with Thomas Harris (no relation), bestselling author of *Silence of the Lambs,* who compared writing to digging a fifty-foot ditch. However, at other times, once I get into it, I start feeling good; I feel inspired, excited and revved up about what I am writing. Thus, the way I feel is largely out of my control; but the action I take is very much within my control.

Adopting the golden rule – action first, feelings later – is a win-win strategy. How so? Because if we're acting on our values, we're creating a richer, fuller life. And if the feelings we want show up later, that's a lovely bonus; after all, we all like to have good feelings. But even if those feelings *don't* show up later – and there's no guarantee they will – we're *still* acting on our values, doing what makes our lives meaningful.

Now take ten seconds and notice what your mind is saying.

***

Is your mind protesting again? Is it saying: 'What do you mean, there's no guarantee that those good feelings will show up later?'

Unfortunately, that's just the way it is. To be accurate, the golden rule should be stated like this: *The actions of confidence come first; the feelings of confidence often come later, but not always.* This is simply acknowledging reality: we have far more control over our actions than over our feelings. Our minds don't like to admit this, so don't take my word for it: check it out with this simple thought experiment.

Suppose I held a gun to your head and asked you to do something you've never done before in your life, like juggling flaming torches, riding a unicycle or somersaulting from a flying trapeze; would you do it? For sure you would. You wouldn't do it very well; you'd make lots of mistakes; you might never succeed in balancing on that unicycle, or keeping those torches in the air, or somersaulting from the trapeze – but with a gun at your head, you'd certainly give it a go.

Now suppose I tell you to *feel confident* while you're learning to do those things. Could you do it? No way! And that's why the golden rule is 'actions first'.

DISCIPLINE AND WILLPOWER

The 'no motivation' story has two close relatives: 'I've got no discipline' and 'I've got no willpower.' Our mind can easily hook us with these stories, and turn them into self-fulfilling prophecies. The fantasy our minds conjure up is that there is something called 'discipline' or 'willpower' and once we possess this thing, we'll be able to start doing what really matters. This fantasy is reinforced by everyday language: when we hear, 'It takes discipline to get up early in the morning and go to the gym', it sounds like there is some magic potion called 'discipline', and until we have this magic potion, we can't get up early and go to the gym.

Unfortunately, if we buy into this fantasy, then we encounter one of two problems. Problem one: we go off in search of the magic potion – reading books or doing courses to try and develop more willpower or discipline – instead of committing to action right now.

Problem two: we decide the magic potion is unobtainable, and we give up on doing what matters because we 'don't have enough' discipline or willpower.

So let's be clear: there is no magic potion; there is no chemical, hormone, gene or part of the brain called 'discipline' or 'willpower'. These words are merely descriptive labels; they are ways of describing a pattern of committed action. When we say someone has discipline or willpower, all we mean is this: this person consistently commits to acting on their values, and doing what is required to achieve their goals – *even when they don't feel like doing it*.

So once again, actions come first, feelings later. First we learn to act consistently on our values, irrespective of how we are feeling. And after we have established that as a habit, then we will feel like we have discipline or willpower.

SNEAKY HOOKS

Our minds will never run out of ways to hook us, and as you can see, some hooks are sneakier than others. These stories about lack of motivation, willpower and discipline are particularly seductive, but they are all basically variants of 'I can't do it; I'm not good enough.'

So next time you hear your mind say, 'I've got no motivation', recognize that's actually impossible and unhook yourself. Then clarify the desire that is driving your behaviour. Is it the desire to avoid discomfort and do what makes you feel good in the short term (avoidance drive)? Or is it the desire to act on your values and do what enriches your life in the long term (values drive)?

Next ask yourself, 'If I let this desire dictate my actions, will it take my life in the direction I want to go?'

Finally ask yourself, 'Even though I don't feel motivated, am I willing to do what will make my life richer?'

And if you answer yes, then ACT: accept your thoughts and feelings, choose a valued direction, take action mindfully.

However, if your answer is no, then you'll need to unleash ...

chapter 20

the power of self-acceptance

Michael Jordan's biography, on the website of the National Basketball Association, reads: 'By acclamation, Michael Jordan is the greatest basketball player of all time.'

It's hard to believe that at the age of sixteen, he failed to make it into his high school basketball team. But it's not so hard to believe that he practised long and hard and made it into the team the following year. Jordan has a healthy attitude towards failure, taking the view that in learning to do anything well, we're going to make plenty of mistakes along the way. And the further we venture into uncharted waters, the more likely we are to screw up.

Now, I don't know anybody who *likes* making mistakes or screwing up, but if we can accept failure as an essential part of all self-development, we'll be much better off than if we fight it. Many successful people have spoken on this subject. Thomas Watson, president of IBM, was asked, 'What is the formula for success?' He replied: 'Double your rate of failure.'

The great wartime leader Sir Winston Churchill said: 'Success is the ability to go from failure to failure without loss of enthusiasm.'

And the US philosopher John Dewey put it this way: 'Failure is instructive. The person who really thinks learns quite as much from his failures as from his successes.'

But while it's easy to go along with this intellectually, it's hard to actually embrace it in reality. Why? Because failure does not feel good! Earlier I mentioned 'the reality gap': that painful gap between the reality we want and the reality we've actually got. The bigger the reality gap, the more painful the feelings that arise. And failure pulls us smack-bang into that gap. And that hurts, badly. For most of us, it hurts every bit as much as a physical injury – if not more so. No wonder we all tend to fear it!

Now, as you know, human beings do not like uncomfortable feelings. So to avoid the pain of failure, we often quit, or give up before we get started. And instead we do something easier, something less challenging. And very often, this will give us a feeling of relief. But it doesn't last. Before long, our minds start beating us up for 'quitting', or we feel that sense of heaviness, loss and stagnation that characterizes life inside the 'comfort zone'.

So what are we to do?

CHANGING OUR RELATIONSHIP WITH FAILURE

There are at least three ways I know of to transform our relationship with failure. The first is by regularly reminding ourselves that failure is a fact of life. To help with this, it's useful to collect relevant stories. For example:

- Walt Disney's first animation studio, 'Iwerks-Disney Commercial Artists', went bust after just one month.
- Oprah Winfrey lost her job as news anchor on WJZ-TV in Baltimore. They told her that she 'wasn't fit for television'.

- Albert Einstein wanted to attend the prestigious Swiss Polytechnic Institute, but he did not pass the entrance examination.
- Steven Spielberg applied to the University of Southern California School of Theater, Film and Television on three separate occasions – but each time he was unsuccessful because of his C grade average.
- The first business venture of Microsoft co-founders Bill Gates and Paul Allen was called 'Traf-O-Data'. It analysed traffic flow – and it flopped miserably.
- Abraham Lincoln was defeated in his first bid for a seat in the Illinois House of Representatives. He then opened a general store, but within a few months, it went under.

Collecting favourite quotes can also be helpful. Here are two I especially like, because they're so relevant to writers:

'Writing is being prepared to be stupid and make mistakes.' Peter Carey, internationally bestselling author

'The first draft of anything is shit.' Ernest Hemingway, one of the greatest writers of the twentieth century

When I'm slogging away at my computer, and my mind's telling me that everything I write is terrible, I always come back to these two quotes; I give myself permission to be stupid, to make mistakes, and to produce shit. I defuse from the tyrannical dictator inside my head who insists that everything I write has to be good. And I remind myself that it's only the first draft, and with each edit and rewrite it will get better.

The second approach is to think of failure as nothing more

than honest feedback. When we fail at something, it is simply feedback that what we are doing isn't working. This was Thomas Edison's attitude when working on the light bulb. After years of unsuccessful experiments in which light bulb after light bulb exploded, fizzled out or never got started, he famously said, 'I haven't failed; I've just found 10,000 ways that won't work.'

With this attitude, we can more readily remember that failure is a natural part of learning. It's an opportunity to reflect on what didn't work, and to think about what might work better next time. In the words of Henry Ford: 'Failure provides the opportunity to begin again, more intelligently.'

The third approach is to play by the rule discussed in chapter 12:

Rule 6: True success means living by your values.

Playing the game this way means that as long as I've acted on my values, then even if I don't achieve my goal, I am still successful.

For example, I have four unpublished novels sitting in my drawers. From a goal-focused viewpoint, these are all failures, because I haven't succeeded in my goal of getting them published. But from a values-focused perspective, they are all successes, because in every moment of writing, I have lived by my values around creativity, self-expression and personal growth.

And then there's the one novel I *have* had published: a sex comedy called *Stand Up Strummer.* Despite some good reviews (one newspaper called it 'Bridget Jones for blokes') the book didn't sell very well. So does the fact that it got published make it a success? Or does the fact that it didn't sell well make it a failure? From a values-focused perspective, such questions are irrelevant. The important fact is this: I lived my values and found the process challenging, rewarding and fulfilling. To me, that *is* success. (Of course,

I was disappointed with the ultimate outcome. I'd have loved it to be a huge international bestseller, and get made into a Hollywood movie starring Colin Firth and Renee Zellweger. But as the great guru Mick Jagger so famously sang: 'You can't always get what you want.')

REBOUNDING FROM FAILURE

When we get stuck, screw up, fail, make mistakes or go off track, our minds like to pull out a stick and clobber us. They may even insist that beating ourselves up is a good thing to do: 'That will teach you'; 'You have to be tough with yourself!' So let me ask you: if beating yourself up were a good way to change behaviour, wouldn't you be perfect by now? After all, how many hidings have you given yourself over the years? Did they lead to lasting, healthy change?

You probably know the old saying: if you want to get your donkey to carry your load, you can use either a carrot or a stick. In other words, you can beat it with a stick until it grudgingly goes along with your wishes, or you can dangle a fresh juicy carrot in front of it, and once it's carried your load to where you want, you give it the carrot as a reward. Both approaches will get your donkey moving. However, if you always rely on the stick, you'll soon have a miserable, unhealthy donkey. Conversely, if you rely on the carrot, you'll end up with a healthy, happy donkey (who also has excellent night vision).

The human mind has quite a range of sticks; does yours use any of the following: 'Idiot!', 'Loser!', 'Quitter!', 'I knew this would happen', 'How could I be so stupid?', 'I'll never get it right', 'This just proves how inadequate I am', 'It's not fair; this doesn't happen to other people', 'There's something wrong with me!', 'I'm useless', 'Why is it so hard?', 'Stupid! Stupid! Stupid!', 'I can't believe I did that', 'Why does this keep happening to me?', 'I just don't have what it takes', 'What a waste of time', 'I'm weak', 'I never should have bothered', 'The whole idea was crazy; it was doomed to fail from the beginning', 'I'm hopeless'?

Sometimes our minds even turn that stick on to others, and we get all caught up in the blame game: 'This would never have happened if he/she/they hadn't done what they did. It's their fault!' But wherever the blows land, on us or others, one thing's for sure: they don't help us to accept the pain of failure, or to learn and grow from the experience.

THE ART OF REBOUNDING FROM FAILURE

There are six basic steps for rebounding from failure.

Step 1: Unhook

Notice, name and neutralize your mind's harsh commentary. Say to yourself, 'Aha! It's clobbering time!', or 'Oho! The "loser" story again!', or 'I'm noticing my mind beating up on me', or 'I'm having the thought that I failed miserably.' Let those thoughts come and go like passing cars, let Radio Failure blast in the background, thank your mind for its comments, and engage fully in whatever you are doing.

Step 2: Make room

Expand around the pain. Observe those painful sensations in your body, breathe into them, and open up around them. And if you're somewhere private, you may like to place a hand on where it hurts most, and 'hold the pain gently'. (Over the years, I've worked with many 'tough guys' such as cops, firemen, soldiers and elite athletes who initially baulked at the idea of doing this – it seemed effeminate or too 'touchy-feely' to them – and yet almost all of them, once they had gotten over their reluctance, found it very helpful.)

Step 3: Be kind

If you come down on yourself like a ton of bricks, it will not give you health and vitality in the long term. You'll end up like that battered, miserable donkey. And the macho 'suck it up' attitudes so common in the sporting and business worlds simply do not sustain most people in the long term. True mental toughness – the ability to persist in your endeavour, despite great pain – develops through self-acceptance, kindness to yourself, and the ongoing commitment to acting on core values. So if you want to rebound and thrive after failure, you need to be kind to yourself.

Imagine that someone you love was feeling what you are feeling under similar circumstances; how would you treat them? If you point the finger and judge them – 'You need to try harder', 'Pull your finger out', 'Don't be a wimp', 'You've only got yourself to blame' – then not only will that person feel worse, but your harsh, judgemental response will damage the relationship.

On the other hand, if you rush in and try to fix it with positive thinking – 'No use crying over spilt milk', 'Every cloud has a silver lining', 'One door opens and another closes', 'Rome wasn't built in a day', 'What doesn't kill you makes you stronger' – the other person is likely to feel irritated, sad or disappointed. Why? Because this 'super-positive, fix-it-up, make-it-right and get-over-it' attitude lacks empathy and compassion; such an attitude suggests that you either don't understand or don't care how much the other person is hurting.

So if you wanted to treat this other person with respect, kindness and compassion, while genuinely acknowledging just how painful failure is, then what kind and considerate words would you say to them? If you're struggling for ideas, here's one possibility: 'I know when things like this happen, it hurts like hell. I wish I could take your pain away, but I know that's not possible. I just want you to know I'm here for you.' Try saying something similar to yourself – with *genuine* kindness. And also consider: is there something kind or compassionate you could do for yourself? (Hint: placing a hand on the pain, as in step 2, is a strong gesture of compassion towards yourself.)

Step 4: Appreciate what worked

An important act of kindness towards yourself is to acknowledge and appreciate everything you did that worked. No matter how poorly you played the game or performed in the interview, painted the canvas or handled your kids, there were undoubtedly some things you did that were okay, and maybe even some things you did very well. What did you do that was an improvement – no matter how small – on last time? What did you do that was reasonable? What did you do that worked well? What did you do that involved taking a risk or trying something new?

Acknowledge and appreciate these efforts, and give yourself a pat on the back for what you did right. This is absolutely essential for self-encouragement. It's not enough to merely unhook from all our harsh criticisms and self-judgements; we need to actively appreciate our efforts, especially when we fail to achieve our goals. Each time we do this, we are learning how to be an effective coach. Ineffective coaches focus only on what went wrong, and do so in a harsh, judgemental manner. Effective coaches first acknowledge and appreciate what went right – and then, in a respectful, non-judgemental manner, they acknowledge what went wrong and turn it into a useful learning experience.

Step 5: Find something useful

Look for something useful in this failure. Ask yourself, 'How can I learn or grow from this?'; 'What could I do differently next time that might lead to a better outcome?' Every failure, no matter what it involves, gives us an opportunity to learn and grow – even if only to improve our defusion and expansion skills. The point is *not* to try to diminish, negate or trivialize the pain of failure, but rather to dignify it and have something beneficial come out of it.

Step 6: Take a stand

Ask yourself, 'What do I want to stand for in the face of this reality gap?' You can stand for giving up, or you can stand for something more life-enhancing. What values would you like to bring into play: persistence, learning, courage, adaptability, innovation, creativity, personal growth or others? Use those values to guide the way you respond. Ask yourself, 'What would I need to do so that ten years from now I could look back with pride and satisfaction in the way I responded?' Then take that action, mindfully.

And if you get stuck, go off track or start running out of steam, then firmly (but kindly and respectfully) remind yourself of the actions you need to take, and why they are important to you. Joe Simpson did this repeatedly throughout his gruelling journey back to base camp. In *Touching the Void,* he referred to this pattern of thinking as 'the voice'. In the midst of all his despairing, hopeless, defeatist thoughts, he would hear 'the voice' reminding him of what he needed to do to survive: Get up, keep moving, don't stop. We can all cultivate an inner voice that kindly, firmly and respectfully reminds us what we need to do: keep practising, keep learning, keep growing.

SIX STEPS FOR REBOUNDING FROM FAILURE
1. Unhook from unhelpful thoughts
2. Make room for painful feelings
3. Be kind to yourself, in word and gesture
4. Acknowledge what worked and appreciate any improvements

5.   Find something useful to help you learn or grow
6.   Take a stand through acting on your values

We now have yet another rule for the confidence game:

Rule 9: Failure hurts – but if we're willing to learn, it's a wonderful teacher.

When playing by this rule, effective self-encouragement is essential: being kind to ourselves, acknowledging what worked, learning and growing from our experience, and reconnecting with our values. Without these steps, failure is merely a weight around our necks. But with good self-encouragement, we can truly appreciate the process of . . .

chapter 21

getting better

'You better get secretarial work or get married.' This is what the director of the Blue Book modelling agency advised the aspiring model Marilyn Monroe in 1944.

'The singer will have to go; the BBC won't like him.' Eric Easton, the first manager of The Rolling Stones, made this comment about Mick Jagger after watching the band perform.

'We don't like their sound, and guitar music is on the way out.' This was the verdict from Decca Recording Co when they rejected The Beatles in 1962.

'It will be years – not in my time – before a woman will become prime minister.' Margaret Thatcher said this in 1974, five years before she became prime minister of Britain.

★★★

What all these comments show is that we can't predict the future. We don't know what is possible. With persistence, courage and the willingness to learn and grow, we are often capable of achieving far more than anyone – including ourselves – might ever have expected.

Now I don't want to turn into a motivational guru and start telling you that 'You can achieve anything you want if only you put your mind to it.' Such statements are, in my opinion, ridiculous. But I do invite you to consider something very carefully. Throughout this book, I've mentioned many inspiring people. And while they all had different visions, goals and action plans, they all shared (at least) two core values: persistence and self-development.

Persistence is the quality of continuing resolutely, despite problems or difficulties.

Self-development is the quality of working to improve, strengthen or advance your skills and abilities.

If we choose to live by these values, we will reap many rewards. We might not achieve all our goals, or make all our dreams come true, but we will improve significantly at doing what matters to us.

I started writing books when I was twenty-three, and by the time I was thirty-nine I had written five – and all were unpublished. My sixth book, *The Happiness Trap*, was published shortly after my fortieth birthday. What kept me going through the dark patches, through those times when I felt lost, dispirited or too tired to carry on, were my values around persistence and self-development. Even today, with four published books under my belt, I still get hooked by my mind's judgements that what I'm writing is boring or unoriginal, or by its predictions that 'This book will be a flop.' At other times I hit a wall, run out of ideas, or get totally stuck for words. When this happens, I turn to my values to get me through. I ask myself, 'Do I value developing my writing skills further? Do I value persisting in the face of obstacles?'

The answer to these questions is always 'yes'. (And that in itself gives me a little buzz; it's usually rewarding when we acknowledge our values.) Then I ask myself, 'So am I willing to keep on writing, even though I don't feel like it, and my mind's telling me it's crap?' Nineteen times out of twenty, the answer is 'yes'. This is enough to get me back at the computer, doing what needs to be done to finish the book. (And one time in twenty, it's not enough – so I go and do something else instead. But at least I am being honest with myself, rather than 'reason-giving'.)

Now pause for ten seconds and notice what your mind is saying.

***

By this point in the book, I am expecting a diverse range of responses. Some minds are probably going 'Yes! Yes! Yes!' Other minds are probably protesting loudly. One of the most common protests is this: 'That's all very well, but I don't have those values. I don't value persistence and self-development.' Well, one of the beautiful things about values is we can choose them, right now, in this moment. So even if for our whole lives, up to this point in time, we have never lived by values such as persistence or self-development, we can choose to start right now. We can persist a little longer than last time; or work even a little at improving the way we do things. (Of course, you don't *have to* choose these values; but if you want the benefits they can bring, then you *can* choose them any time you like.)

Another great thing about values is that they never disappear. They are always there, waiting for us; and in any moment we can act on them, or not. So even if we go off track and forget about our values for weeks, months or years, at any moment we like, we can come back to them. (Remember: that is the secret of instant success!)

When looking at people such as Nelson Mandela, Lance Armstrong, Joe Simpson and Martin Luther King Jr, we could focus on many different values, but I've highlighted persistence and self-development because of their key roles in the confidence game. To quote Calvin Coolidge, thirtieth president of the US: 'Nothing in the world can take the place of persistence. Talent will not; nothing is more common than unsuccessful men with talent. Genius will not; unrewarded genius is almost a proverb. Education will not; the world is full of educated derelicts. Persistence and determination are omnipotent. The slogan "press on" has solved and always will solve the problems of the human race.'

IMPORTANT VALUES

A quick refresher: the five main causes of low self-confidence are excessive expectations, harsh self-judgement, preoccupation with fear, lack of experience and lack of skills. So if your skills are already well developed, and more than adequate for the demands of the tasks you face, then your low self-confidence lies in the other four areas. However, if your skills aren't up to the demands of the task, then clearly you will need to work on them. So let's take one final look at that Confidence Cycle.

I've lost track of how many times I've said it now (so please feel free to scream if I'm driving you crazy): if we want to be good at something, we have to practise. And naturally, given that we are all busy people, and practice not only takes time but brings up discomfort, most of us have a tendency to avoid it. This is where the values of persistence and self-development are so useful. By connecting with these values, we can get ourselves moving in the right direction, even when we don't feel like it. We can remind ourselves:

THE CONFIDENCE CYCLE
(or how to get good at doing anything)

1. Practise the skills
2. Apply them effectively
3. Assess the results
4. Modify as needed

'Here's an opportunity for self-development.' Or we can say to ourselves, 'Persistence is the key!'

Obviously you don't have to use these precise words. A more common term for self-development is 'personal growth' and more common terms for persistence are 'dedication', 'commitment', 'determination', 'giving it your all', 'going the extra mile', and so on.

While practice is vitally important, it's not enough; we also need to apply our skills effectively. That means we need to make room for our feelings, unhook ourselves from our thoughts and engage fully in the task at hand.

Finally, once we've done that, we need to assess the results and modify our actions as needs. This is easily said and done, but to do it well we require . . .

SELF-AWARENESS

There are three essential elements for self-awareness:

1. Mindfulness
2. Reflection
3. Feedback

Let's quickly go through these.

Mindfulness

If we want to learn and improve, we need to become aware of our habitual patterns of thinking, feeling and acting. Mindfulness enables us to do this. Instead of wandering around on autopilot, we notice with curiosity the stories our minds like to tell us, the feelings that arise when we face challenges, and our habitual patterns of action. The more access we have to this information, the easier change becomes.

Reflection

Mindful awareness of our thoughts, feelings and actions gives us valuable data to work with. The next step is to examine our actions in terms of 'workability': to assess whether what we are doing is working to help us create the lives we want. And we want to do this as non-judgementally as possible. Judging ourselves or our performance as 'pathetic', 'appalling', 'incompetent' or 'useless' will not help us learn and grow; it merely demoralizes us. We can't stop our minds from generating all those harsh judgements and criticisms – that's one of the many things they like to do – but we can repeatedly unhook ourselves and let those thoughts come and go like passing cars.

To develop your ability for self-reflection, get into the habit of asking yourself three simple questions:

- What did I do that worked?
- What did I do that didn't work?
- What could I do differently next time around?

Feedback

Mindfulness and self-reflection can only get us so far. For maximal self-awareness we need feedback from others. But we don't want any old feedback; ideally we want feedback that is honest, practical and non-judgemental, delivered by trustworthy and competent others. This is why every top athlete has a coach.

Honesty is vitally important. If the feedback we get is exaggeratedly positive *or* exaggeratedly negative, it's not much use. I'm sure you know these two clichés from books, movies or TV: there's the tyrannical executive, surrounded by yes-men who tell him every decision he makes is absolutely wonderful; and there's the humble, dedicated worker who is repeatedly criticized and devalued by an insecure rival. These situations really do exist – they have become clichés because they are so common in the workplace – and they are recipes for disaster. We need honest, non-judgemental feedback from people we can trust about what is working, what is not working, and what can be done differently. And we want it from people who are competent to give it: people who have enough skills, information and experience to know what they are talking about.

So if we are aiming to improve in our chosen field – creative, sporting, business, parenting, social or other – it is advisable to find trustworthy and competent mentors, coaches or advisers; people who can observe and reflect on what we do, and give us useful feedback. This can be confronting or painful, but if it is delivered honestly, respectfully, compassionately and non-judgementally, it is invaluable.

We can also look for what's useful in 'unsolicited feedback'. In other words, when someone abuses, insults or judges us, it's worth looking to see if there's a grain of truth in their words. For example, over the years, quite a few people have called me arrogant (especially my wife). I used to deny it, discount it, or counter-attack with a criticism about the other person (I won't tell you what I called my wife). These days, I usually respond differently (alas, not always); I tend to pause, notice and reflect, considering whether there is something valid in the criticism; to look with openness and curiosity at the way I've been behaving. And if the criticism is valid, I consider: what's working, what's not working, and what could I do differently? Finally I (often, but not always) respond mindfully, acting on my values – which usually means apologizing for my arrogance and expressing myself more respectfully.

SELF-AWARENESS AND SELF-DOUBT

Self-awareness plays a particularly important role in overcoming self-doubt. Suppose Radio Triple F is constantly broadcasting our flaws – 'I'm incompetent', 'I'm boring', 'I'm uncoordinated', 'I'm a lousy player', 'I'm not cut out for this job', 'I'm so unoriginal', 'I'm a fraud', 'No one likes me', 'I've got no talent', 'I can't tell jokes' and so on; how can we tell if we genuinely lack the necessary skills, or if our minds are just doing a hatchet job?

This is a particularly important question when it comes to social confidence. As I mentioned in chapter 10, most people with significant social anxiety do *not* lack social skills. The problem is they are so fused with negative self-judgements ('I'm so dull/ boring/stupid/unlikeable') or harsh self-criticism ('Oh, that came out wrong! Why did I say that?'), and so busy struggling with their feelings of anxiety that they fail to engage fully in the social interaction. This leads to two major problems. Firstly, a lack of fulfilment in socializing: we won't enjoy it if we're not fully present. Secondly, a lack of reliable data about how we are actually performing: if we're not mindfully engaged, if we're all caught up in the ongoing commentary inside our head, then we can't accurately read others' responses.

The same issues arise in 'impostor syndrome' or any other form of pervasive self-doubt. Yes, unhooking from our mind's judgements is important, but not enough in itself; developing self-awareness is essential. In other words, we need to:

1. Mindfully engage in the task at hand.
2. Later reflect on what we have directly observed (as opposed to buying into our mind's commentary on what occurred).
3. If still in doubt, get honest, non-judgemental feedback from trusted, competent others.

BETTER OR BEST?

In this chapter we've focused on improving, advancing and getting better. And in many areas of life, we may be happy to let this happen at its own pace; as long as we know we're learning, growing and developing, we're not driven to excel. For example, while I want to become competent at riding my bicycle, I have no inclination to try to excel at it. Similarly, I want to get better at lifting weights in the gym, but I am not in the least bit interested in trying to excel at it. However, for most of us, there are at least one or two areas of life in which we *do* want to push ourselves; where it's not enough to simply get better, we want to do the best we possibly can.

Now before we go any further, I wish to declare loudly: I do *not* recommend taking this attitude to every area of your life! If you're always trying to do your very best at everything, you've been hooked by perfectionism. Motivational gurus love to shout from the rooftops, 'Always do your best! Always give one hundred per cent!', but if we follow this rule, it's a recipe for major stress and burnout. Lance Armstrong knew that if he trained as hard as possible all year round, he would not reach his peak; he knew the importance of giving himself 'down time'. So for several months of the year, he would deliberately ease off the pressure: cut down significantly on his training, increase the amount of fun and play in his life, and avoid entering major competitions. We can all learn from this.

So, keeping this caution in mind, if you want to be the best parent, partner, lover, businessperson, entrepreneur, artist, musician or athlete that you can be; if you wish to perform that role to the best of your ability, then think about what it takes to . . .

chapter 22

reach the peak

He speaks from the heart: genuine, open, enthusiastic. His words flow spontaneously as he reaches out to each and every member of the audience.

She leaps through the air like a panther, oblivious to the crowd of spectators. In one smooth motion, she lifts, aims and shoots. The ball flies across the court and into the basket.

His fingers have become one with the piano keys. Enraptured by the melody, the music seems to well from within his soul.

She is so absorbed in the conversation that when she eventually looks at her watch, she is shocked to find that two hours have passed.

★★★

Athletes call it 'being in the zone'; psychologists call it 'flow'. It is a state of total absorption in the task at hand. Our focus is narrowed; time seems to stop; there is no self-consciousness, no internal commentary on our performance; nothing distracts us; our attention is completely on the task; all those skills we've practised come together so fluidly that action seems effortless; our bodies and minds work together in perfect harmony. It is in this state that peak performance happens. This gives us our final rule for the confidence game:

Rule 10: The key to peak performance is total engagement in the task.

THE THREE PHASES OF PERFORMANCE

In their excellent book *The Psychology of Enhancing Human Performance* psychologists Frank Gardner and Zella Moore describe three phases of performance: the pre-performance phase, the performance phase, and the post-performance response phase. As you read on, keep in mind that when it comes to sport, business and stage performance, these three phases are easy to distinguish, but when it comes to performance in other domains of life such as parenting, painting, socializing or writing books, the phases are not so distinct; they do exist, but they blur into one another.

The pre-performance phase

This phase is all about preparation, training and practice. This is where we read books, attend training and practise our essential skills (especially mindfulness skills). We'll need to come back repeatedly to our values – especially self-development and persistence; defuse from all those reasons not to practise; make room for the discomfort that's involved; and engage fully in practising the skills we need.

The performance phase

This is where it all comes together: where we apply the skills effectively in the performance situation. The key here is 'task-focused attention'. In other words, our attention must be focused on whatever is essential to do the task well. Whether we're kicking a ball, writing a book, chairing a meeting, sharing ideas, making love, playing with our kids, painting a portrait, strumming a guitar, or giving a speech, the spotlight needs to shine only on what is relevant for successful action.

Here are a few things that definitely should not be in the spotlight: thoughts about what you look like; thoughts about what others are thinking; thoughts about how to move and where to put your arms, legs, mouth and head; thoughts about how well or poorly you're doing; thoughts about what the ultimate outcome will be; thoughts about what might happen five minutes from now; thoughts about what happened five minutes ago; thoughts about what you could be doing better; thoughts about failure; thoughts about success; thoughts about mindfulness; thoughts about how you are feeling; thoughts about the mistakes you've made; thoughts about your strengths; thoughts about your weaknesses; thoughts about how others will judge your performance; thoughts about what might go wrong; and so on and so on.

These thoughts, and many others, do nothing more than distract us from the task at hand. But knowing this intellectually and telling ourselves not to have such thoughts will not stop them from appearing. (If you don't believe me, try it.) And if we start challenging these thoughts, or trying to push them away, or reciting positive affirmations, then all we are doing is creating further distractions instead of focusing attention on the task at hand.

So what are we to do? This is where we require all our mindfulness skills: defusion from unhelpful thoughts, expansion around difficult feelings, and total engagement in the task-relevant aspects of our experience. As elite cricketer Justin Langer describes it in his book *Seeing the Sunrise*: 'As a batsman, at the moment the bowler lets go of the ball, my mind must be completely focused on *that ball* and nothing else.'

While we can't eliminate unhelpful thoughts and difficult feelings, we can make space for them while remaining focused and engaged in what we are doing. And the greater our ability to do this, the better our performance.

Only once our skills are sufficiently developed to meet the demands of the situation can we expect to enter 'the zone', or a state of 'flow'. If we don't have adequate skills, naturally we will struggle. However, we shouldn't try to force a state of flow; the very effort to do so usually prevents it. (After all, if we're getting caught up in thoughts like, 'I have to get into the zone' or 'How do I get into a state of flow?', then clearly we're not engaging fully in the task.)

Flow states arise spontaneously under two conditions: a) our skills are good enough for the task; b) we engage fully in what we are doing. It is in these states of mindful, focused action that humans perform at their peak: the golfer melds with the golf club; the singer becomes one with the audience; the words flow effortlessly from the writer; and the boxer floats like a butterfly, stings like a bee.

The post-performance response phase

How we respond *after* our performance is just as important as what happens before and during it. Regardless of how well or poorly we did, the healthiest attitude is to reflect mindfully on our performance, and learn and grow from it. Can we bring an attitude of openness and curiosity as we reflect on the three questions: what worked, what didn't work, and what could we do differently next time?

If we are pleased with our performance, let's thoroughly celebrate and congratulate ourselves for all our hard work (while being careful not to fuse with 'I am the greatest!'). If our performance didn't meet our expectations, we need to practise self-acceptance: defuse from harsh self-judgements, speak to ourselves kindly, come back to our values, and commit to learning and growing from the experience. For most of us, this doesn't come naturally. When our minds start to criticize, we are easily hooked. Still, the moment that we realize we've been hooked, we can unhook ourselves and re-engage in the present.

Finally, everyone likes to be appreciated, so let's make sure that we actively appreciate ourselves. Appreciate your commitment, appreciate everything you did that worked reasonably well, appreciate your own willingness to take a risk, and especially appreciate *anything* you did that was an improvement on last time, no matter how small it may be. This is essential, not only for self-acceptance, but also for ongoing energy, drive and enthusiasm.

***

Hopefully you can see how all three phases of performance require us to play by the golden rule: *The actions of confidence come first; the feelings of confidence come later.*

The more we take the actions of confidence – the more we rely on ourselves to do the training, practise the skills, develop our mindfulness, step out of the comfort zone, face our challenges and learn from our failures – the more our performance improves. And the better our performance, the more likely we are to *feel* confident. But if we try to do things the other way around, to wait until we feel confident *before* we take action, it clearly won't work.

And it's worth a reminder that even when we do feel confident, that does not mean an absence of fear. No matter how skilled and accomplished we are, when we face a genuine challenge where something important is at stake, the fight-or-flight response will kick in.

FINDING A HEALTHY BALANCE

Read the sports section of any newspaper and you'll soon find stories of injured athletes. Often these stories applaud the athlete's heroic ability to play on despite intense pain. A classic example was Tiger Woods' stellar performance in the 2008 US Open: despite pain in his left knee, on which he had already had arthroscopic surgery on two previous occasions, he managed to win the tournament. This prompted his competitor, Kenny Perry, to comment that 'He beat everybody on one leg.'

In a similar vein, earlier in this book, I praised Joe Simpson's persistence and ability to focus on the task despite the agonizing pain from his shattered leg. But we have to be careful; there is a dark side to this ability. Many athletes get so focused on achieving their goals that they fail to pay attention to their bodies. As a result, they may unnecessarily injure themselves, make the injury worse, or delay recovery by prematurely returning to the game instead of allowing time for proper healing.

We see the same thing in the business world: the high-flyer who dedicates himself to work and achieves astonishing results but eventually comes crashing down with depression, addiction or a stress-related medical condition such as high blood pressure (or even a heart attack).

We also see this happening with artists, writers, dancers, musicians and performers of all kinds: they are so extremely focused on achieving results that they neglect their own health and wellbeing. This cannot be sustained indefinitely; over time it is guaranteed to lead to burnout, injury or illness.

To sustain peak performance in the long term, there are no two ways about it: we have to look after our health and wellbeing. And that means not only taking care of our bodies, but also our relationships. Sadly, the world of 'high achievers' is not only full of stress-related illness, but also heartbreak, divorce and broken families. Does it have to be this way?

Naturally, excellence requires sacrifice. That's a given. If we want to excel at anything – parenting, sport, music, speaking, writing, selling, cooking or ballet dancing – then we'll need to make it a priority. We'll need to devote time, energy and effort to it. And that means we'll have to make sacrifices; we'll have to give up doing other things that compete for our time and energy. But we need to be smart about what we sacrifice. To give up watching crappy late-night television is probably wise. But to give up spending quality time with our kids . . . well, I don't need to spell it out, do I? An extreme focus on any endeavour, to the exclusion of all else, often gives fantastic results in that domain of life, but if our loved ones get neglected or hurt in the process, is the sacrifice worth it?

There is no simple solution to this issue. We need to make time to reflect on some difficult questions. The first question is this: in this area of my life, am I content to be competent, or is it truly important for me to excel? Most of us can find great fulfilment in being competent, while also living a balanced and rewarding life. However, many of us will at some point find an area of life where we want to go beyond competence; where we want to do our best to truly excel. (For example, I want to excel at parenting, and I want to excel at writing – and I have plenty of work to do in both areas.) The thing is, as I mentioned earlier, if we want to excel at something it almost always requires significant sacrifice over a long period of time. So you have to ask yourself: what are you willing to give up, and is it worth it? Only you can answer that question. (But please reflect on it carefully and don't buy into the pithy catchphrases of motivational gurus who tell you that you always have to do your very best, always strive for excellence, always give 100 per cent; if you follow such advice blindly, you're heading for misery and burnout.)

The challenge we all face is to find the best possible balance between love, work and play, while staying mindful of our health and wellbeing. And none of us will get it perfectly right. But if we take the time to check in regularly, we can certainly improve it.

So why not try this for yourself? Once a week, take five minutes to reflect honestly on how you're faring in love, work, play and health. Are you living by your values in each area? Is there any room for improvement or adjusting the balance? You could mark it in your calendar or diary; perhaps call it the 'weekly check-up'. You could even discuss it with your partner or a trusted friend.

I know all too well from personal experience that it's easy to dismiss this advice. Our minds seduce us with the story that *after* we finally achieve our big goal, *then* we can get some balance in our lives. Unfortunately, this is rarely the case. Once that goal is achieved, another one rears its head almost immediately. Nelson Mandela put it this way: 'After climbing a great hill, one only finds that there are many more hills to climb.' In other words . . .

chapter 23

it ain't over till it's over

'Making your mark on the world is hard. If it were easy, everybody would do it. But it's not. It takes patience, it takes commitment, and it comes with plenty of failure along the way. The real test is not whether you avoid this failure, because you won't. It's whether you let it harden or shame you into inaction, or whether you learn from it; whether you choose to persevere.' Barack Obama

I don't know about you, but I love self-help books where the author admits to their own imperfections. It makes me feel like a normal human being. From time to time I read a book by someone who claims to have overcome all their mental obstacles, who never gets stuck, who never falls short of their ideals. This seems so far removed from normal human experience, it's hard for me to give it any credit. Maybe there are some perfect human beings out there – but I doubt it.

So, confession time: I've been living and breathing ACT for years now: writing about it, teaching it, practising it. And it has helped me enormously in my own life. And yet, at times I forget almost everything I've written in this book. At times I get hooked by the 'I can't do it' or the 'I'm not good enough' story. At times I go into avoidance mode. At times I lose touch with my values, fail to follow through on my commitments, and act in self-defeating ways. Why? Because I'm a normal human being: fallible and imperfect. Just like you. And this will happen to all of us. Repeatedly.

Personally, my biggest ongoing challenge is in the realm of health. In my early twenties, I was not only obese but dangerously unfit, to the extent of having mild high blood pressure. In my mid-twenties, I started taking better care of myself: exercising and being more sensible about what I ate, and slimming down to a healthy body weight. While I have never gone back to being overweight or dangerously unfit, I do periodically backslide to some degree. There are periods where I eat very healthily, exercise regularly and get myself trim and terrific. And there are other periods where I stop exercising, stuff my face with chocolate, cookies and ice-cream, and pile on the weight again. And then I recognize that I've gone off track, and get back on track again. And so on and so on. This isn't ideal; there's obviously plenty of room for improvement; but beating myself up about it will not help me.

The fact is, no matter how good we get at mindful, values-based living – even if we become Zen masters – there will be times that we forget. We'll fall back into old habits, we'll act in self-defeating ways, and we will hurt and suffer as a result.

Our minds don't want to accept this. Our minds want us to become perfect; to eliminate all our 'flaws' and 'weaknesses'. And they're quick to beat us up when this doesn't happen. But reality doesn't cater to the wishes of our minds. Perfection may exist in the world of fantasy, of superheroes, magical beings and gods. But it doesn't exist down here on earth.

So should we give up?

No way! Although we'll never be perfect, we can keep on learning and growing until the day we die. We can grow smarter, wiser, more mindful; live more in tune with our values; and get better at taking action when we don't feel like it. In other words, we can continually develop our psychological flexibility: the ability to take effective action, guided by values, with awareness, openness and focus.

We can also develop more self-acceptance and compassion for ourselves, for all those times when we screw up, fail or get hurt. And no matter how many times we go off track . . .

WE CAN ALWAYS START AGAIN (AND AGAIN)

Although I've mentioned Lance Armstrong a lot in this book, I don't agree with everything he says. For example, one of his most famous quotes is this: 'Pain is temporary. Quitting lasts for ever.' While the first sentence is true – pain *is* temporary – the second sentence is false. Quitting lasts only until such time as we once again commit to acting on our values.

That's why, in ACT, we don't spout perfectionist slogans like 'never quit', 'never give up', 'always do your best'. They sound good in theory, but in reality, no human can possibly live up to these ideals. The philosopher Haridas Chaudhuri said it succinctly: 'The greater the emphasis on perfection, the further it recedes.'

In ACT, we encourage acceptance of the reality that we're all imperfect – and yes, there *will* be times that we quit, give up, or get lost. And at the same time we also encourage commitment: to get better at staying on track for longer periods, better at catching ourselves when we go off course, and better at starting again from where we are. In other words, to practise ACT, we:

A – Accept our thoughts and feelings.
C – Choose a valued direction.
T – Take action mindfully.

EVERYTHING TAKES TIME

Rome wasn't built in a day, and confidence doesn't develop overnight. However, you now have everything you need for your ongoing journey. You know the five main reasons for low self-confidence:

1. Excessive expectations
2. Harsh self-judgement
3. Preoccupation with fear
4. Lack of experience
5. Lack of skills

And you also know the solutions:

1. Unhook from excessive expectations
2. Practise self-acceptance and self-encouragement
3. Make room for fear – and, if possible, use it
4. Step out of your comfort zone and get the experience you require
5. Practise the skills, apply them effectively, assess the results, modify as needed

This approach will give you what I call 'genuine confidence'. Genuine confidence is not some pleasant feeling that comes and goes, but a personal quality: the ability to rely on yourself, to trust yourself; to be true to yourself; to act on your core values, irrespective of how you are feeling. Genuine confidence can't be gained through listening to a tape or CD; it requires effort and persistence. But then, so does just about everything important in life. So if your mind starts doing its reason-giving routine, thank it for those thoughts and carry on.

Sometimes people think the ACT approach to confidence means 'fake it until you make it'. This is definitely not the case. There is no need to fake anything; you're much better off being real, genuine and authentic. So when you're feeling fear or anxiety, why not honestly acknowledge it, rather than trying to pretend you don't have any? First and foremost, acknowledge it to yourself: 'Here's anxiety' or 'Here's fear'. However, in some situations, you might also choose to acknowledge it to others. Similarly, when you take action, mindfully acting on your values, there is no need to fake anything. You just do what is important to you, and engage fully in what you are doing. And guess what? In each and every moment that you do this, you are already 'making it': instant success!

THE 'RIGHT' RULES

Below I've listed the ten 'right rules' of the confidence game. However, before you read through them, I think a warning is due: rules become dangerous when we follow them rigidly. So please – hold all these rules very lightly! Be flexible with them: bend them, modify them or drop them as required. They are not the Ten Commandments!

Everything in this book is nothing more nor less than a suggestion. I hope there'll be times you choose to apply what you've read, and I expect there'll be plenty of times that you choose to dismiss it. And that's fine by me. (And I hope it's fine by you, too.) I most certainly wouldn't want you to believe something just because I say so. After all, there is no supreme court out there to declare that some rules are 'right' and others are 'wrong'. So test them out for yourself, and see what happens; let your own experience be the judge.

TEN RULES FOR WINNING THE GAME OF CONFIDENCE

1. The actions of confidence come first; the feelings of confidence come later
2. Genuine confidence is not the absence of fear; it is a transformed relationship with fear

3. 'Negative' thoughts are normal. Don't fight them; defuse them
4. Self-acceptance trumps self-esteem
5. True success is living by your values
6. Hold your values lightly, but pursue them vigorously
7. Don't obsess about the outcome; get passionate about the process
8. Don't fight your fear: allow it, befriend it, and channel it
9. Failure hurts – but if we're willing to learn, it's a wonderful teacher
10. The key to peak performance is total engagement in the task

So please: hold these rules lightly, revisit them regularly, and use them flexibly. And let's end the book with a look at . . .

WHAT LIES AHEAD?

Writing a book like this is a constant balancing act. On the one hand, I want to encourage you to live the best life you possibly can; on the other hand I want you to be realistic. If you get carried away with 'Yes, I can do anything I want!' then you will feel high as a kite for a while – but, like all high-flying kites, eventually you will come crashing back down to earth. So it's good to go in with your eyes open. Expect your journey to involve ups and downs, highs and lows, pleasure and pain. Expect successes and failures, triumphs and disasters, giant leaps forward and major falls backward. And bear in mind the words of Sir Winston Churchill: 'Success is not final; failure is not fatal; it is the courage to continue that counts.'

Personally, I love the word 'courage'. It comes from the Latin word 'cor', which means 'heart'. Thus courage means we do what's in our hearts; in other words, we act on our values!

And when people act courageously, what's the most common emotion that they feel?

Fear!

So courage is not the absence of fear; it's doing what really matters *despite* our fear. And that neatly brings us full circle back to Helen Keller. You may recall that in the introduction to this book, I gave you one of her most famous sayings. Well, that wasn't actually the full quotation; here it is in its entirety:

> *Security is mostly a superstition. It does not exist in nature, nor do the children of men as a whole experience it. Avoiding danger is no safer in the long run than outright exposure. Life is either a daring adventure, or nothing.*

If we choose to make our lives a daring adventure – to step out of our comfort zone; to grow, explore and face our challenges – then we will feel what people feel on daring adventures. Our hearts will race; our bodies will sweat; our stomachs will churn. Fear will show up in all its different varieties: from anxiety to insecurity, from stress to self-doubt, from 'pumped' to panic. And at times our minds will yell at us: 'Heeeeeellllp. Let me off. I wanna go back. It's all too hard. I can't handle it. I'm not good enough.'

However, if we make room for those feelings, unhook from those thoughts, and engage fully in acting on our values, then we are free. We are free to behave like the person we want to be; free to do the things that truly matter to us; and free to live our lives with genuine confidence.

references

Armstrong, Lance, 2003, *Every Second Counts*, New York: Broadway Books.

Baumeister, Roy F., Jennifer D. Campbell, Joachim I. Krueger and Kathleen D. Vohs, May 2003, 'Does High Self-Esteem Cause Better Performance, Interpersonal Success, Happiness, or Healthier Lifestyles?' *Psychological Science in the Public Interest*, Vol. 4, No. 1, pages 1–44.

Dr Seuss Enterprises, 1990, *Oh, the Places You'll Go!* New York: Random House.

Gardner, Frank L. & Zella E. Moore, 2007, *The Psychology of Enhancing Human Performance: The Mindfulness-Acceptance-Commitment (MAC) Approach*, New York: Springer Publishing.

Harris, Russ, 2008, *The Happiness Trap: How to Stop Struggling and Start Living*, Boston: Trumpeter Books.

Hayes, Steven C., Kirk Strosahl & Kelly G. Wilson, 1999, *Acceptance and Commitment Therapy: An Experiential Approach to Behavior Change*, New York: Guilford.

Jones, G., S. Hanton & A. B. J. Swain, 1994, 'Intensity and interpretation of anxiety symptoms in elite and non-elite sports performers', *Personality and Individual Differences*, 17, 657–663.

Jones, G., A. B. J. Swain & L. Hardy, 1993, 'Intensity and direction dimensions of competitive state anxiety and relationships with performance', *Journal of Sport Sciences*, 11, 525–532.

Jones, J. C., T. Bruce & D. H. Barlow, 1986, November, 'The effects of four levels of "anxiety" on sexual arousal in sexually functional and dysfunctional men', Poster session presented at the annual conference of the Association for Advancement of Behavior Therapy, Chicago, Il.

Kashdan, Todd, 2009, *Curious*, New York: HarperCollins.

Langer, Justin, 2008, *Seeing the Sunrise*, Crows Nest NSW, Australia: Allen and Unwin.

Mandela, Nelson Rolihlahla, 1994, *Long Walk to Freedom*, London: Abacus.

Rich, A. R. & D. K. Woolever, 1988, 'Expectancy and self-focused attention: Experimental support for the self-regulation model of test anxiety', *Journal of Social and Clinical Psychology*, 7, 246–259.

Shubin, Neil, 2008, *Your Inner Fish*, London: Penguin Books.

Simpson, Joe, 1988, *Touching the Void*, New York: Harper and Row.

Stengel, Richard, 2008: 'Mandela: His 8 Lessons of Leadership', *Time Magazine*, 9 July 2008.

Swain, A. B. J. & G. Jones, 1996, 'Explaining performance variance: the relative contribution of intensity and direction dimensions of competitive state anxiety', *Anxiety, Stress, and Coping: An International Journal*, 9, 1–18.

Wood, J. V., W. Q. Perunovic & J. W. 2009, July, 'Positive self-statements: power for some, peril for others', *Psychological Science*, 20(7), 860–6.

resources

WORKSHOPS AND TRAINING

Happiness Trap workshops

Russ's Happiness Trap workshops for happiness, confidence and vitality, have been so successful in Australia, he is now introducing them to the UK. Why not come along and amaze yourself at what you are capable of?

ACT is a revolutionary new psychological approach to health, wellbeing and fulfilment. And if you have enjoyed reading *The Confidence Gap*, or *The Happiness Trap*, then you will find these ACT-based workshops transformational. (The difference between the book and the workshop is like the difference between a documentary about Africa and an actual visit to Africa.)

'Happiness Trap' workshops are for everyone, from CEOs to sales staff, from astronauts to homemakers. Whether you're lacking confidence, facing illness, coping with loss, working in a high-stress job, suffering from shyness, struggling with low self-esteem, trying to lose weight or quit smoking, preparing for the biggest challenge of your life, or just wanting to be happier, healthier, and more fulfilled – in the space of just two days, you will learn scientifically proven techniques to:

- Reduce stress and worry
- Rise above fear, doubt and insecurity
- Handle painful thoughts and feelings far more effectively
- Break self-defeating habits
- Develop genuine confidence
- Improve performance and find fulfilment in your work
- Build more satisfying relationships and, above all,
- Create a rich, full and meaningful life.

Russ Harris and his colleagues will start running Happiness Trap workshops in the UK from July 2011. To find out more or enrol in a workshop, go to: www.the happinesstrap.co.uk.

BOOKS BY RUSS HARRIS

The Happiness Trap (Wollongong: Exisle Publishing, 2007)

Many popular notions of happiness are misleading, inaccurate and will actually make you miserable if you believe them. *The Happiness Trap* is a self-help book on how to make life richer, fuller and more meaningful, while avoiding common 'happiness traps'. Based on ACT, it is applicable to everything from work stress to addictions, from anxiety to depression, from the pressures of parenting to the challenges of terminal illness. Used by ACT therapists and their clients all around the world, it is currently translated into fifteen different languages. A website, www.thehappinesstrap.co.uk, offers many free resources to use with the book.

ACT with Love (Oakland: New Harbinger, 2009)

ACT with Love is an inspiring and empowering self-help book that applies the principles of ACT to common relationship issues, and shows how to move from conflict, struggle and disconnection to forgiveness, acceptance, intimacy and genuine loving. It is linked to its own resource-packed website: www.act-with-love.com.

ACT Made Simple (Oakland, CA: New Harbinger, 2009)

A practical and entertaining textbook, ideal for ACT newcomers and experienced ACT professionals alike, ACT Made Simple offers clear explanations of the core ACT processes and a set of real-world tips and solutions for rapidly and effectively implementing them in your coaching or therapy practice. Reading this book is all the training you need to begin using ACT techniques with your clients for impressive results. For more information, visit www.act madesimple.com.

CDS AND MP3S BY RUSS HARRIS

Mindfulness Skills: Volume 1 & Mindfulness Skills: Volume 2

Available as either CDs or downloadable MP3 files, these volumes cover a wide range of mindfulness exercises for personal use. You can order MP3s via www.thehappinesstrap.co.uk. CDs are only available in Australia, and must be ordered through www.actmind fully.com.au.

Online Resources

This book is linked to the website www.thehappinesstrap.co.uk. On this site, on the page titled 'free resources' you can download free copies of the exercises and worksheets in this book. You'll also find some valuable online training in the form of e-courses and webinars.

Newsletter

The *Happiness Trap Newsletter* is a regular, free email newsletter, packed with useful information, tools, and tips relating to ACT. You can register for it under the main menu at any of the websites mentioned above.

acknowledgements

First, a gazillion truckloads of gratitude to my wife, Carmel, for all her love and support; for being my muse; for helping me develop my ideas; for tolerating my love affair with the computer; for looking after our family while I was pounding away at the keyboard; and for encouraging me to keep writing when I was totally convinced it was all 'just a load of crap'.

Also, as usual, a Mount Everest-sized heap of thanks to Steve Hayes, the originator of ACT. And that gratitude also extends to Kelly Wilson and Kirk Strosahl – both huge sources of inspiration for me. Plus a very special thanks to Frank Gardner, whose work on ACT in the realm of peak performance has had a strong influence on my practice. Also to Todd Kashdan, for kindly allowing me to adapt his values worksheet. And a general round of thanks to the larger ACT community worldwide, which is always very supportive; indeed, many ideas within these pages have arisen from discussions on the worldwide ACT Listserv mailing list.

Next I'd like to give a biiiiiiiiiiiiiiigggggggggg 'THANK YOU!' to my agent, Sammie Justesen, for all her good work. Plus I'd like to unload several large shipments of thanks upon the entire team at Penguin – especially Ingrid Ohlsson and Jocelyn Hungerford – for all the hard work, care and attention they have invested in this book.

And finally I want to thank Max – that one special person on this planet who calls me 'Daddy' – simply for bringing so much love, joy and wonder into my life.

index

Note: all exercises in this index are listed in italics.

285